CARUSO'S ME'
VOICE PROD

The Scientific Culture of the Voice

BY

P. MARIO MARAFIOTI, M.D.

PREFACE BY

VICTOR MAUREL

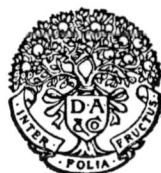

D. APPLETON AND COMPANY

NEW YORK :: 1922 :: LONDON

CARUSO'S METHOD OF VOICE PRODUCTION

The Scientific Culture of the Voice

PRINTED IN THE UNITED STATES OF AMERICA

TO
ENRICO CARUSO
WHOSE SINGING HAS BEEN
THE INSPIRATION OF THIS BOOK

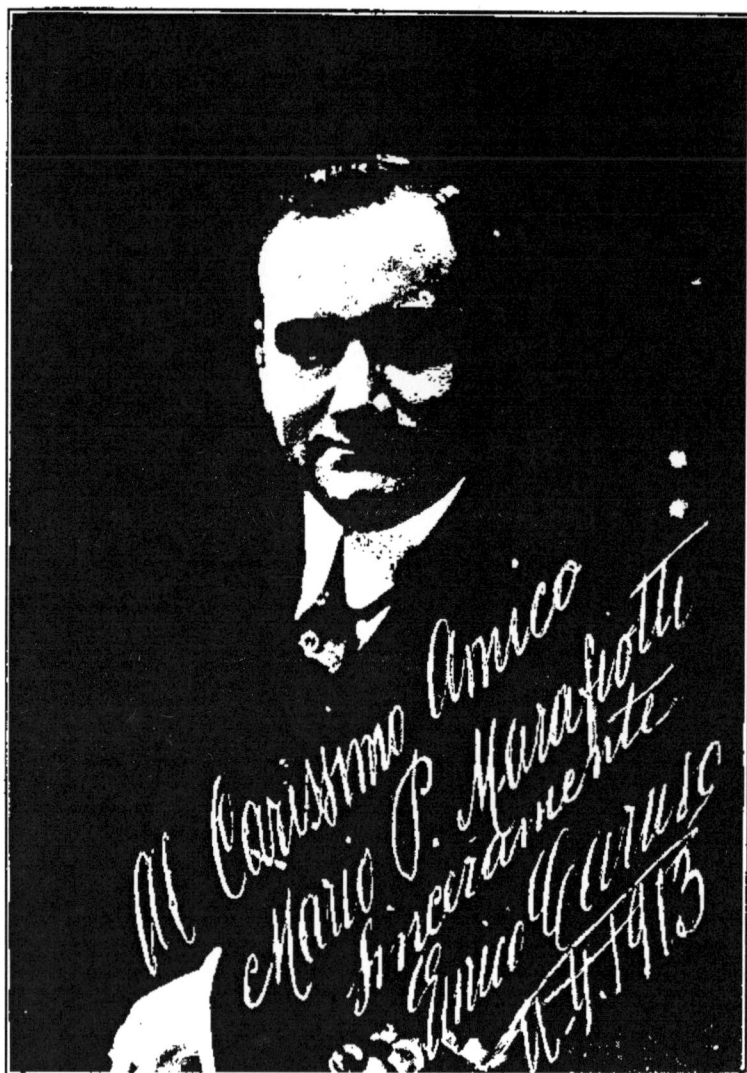

Al Carissimo Amico
Mario P. Marafiotti
Sinceramente
Enrico Caruso
N. Y. 1913

THE CONDADO-VANDERBILT HOTEL
SAN JUAN, PORTO RICO

The VANDERBILT Hotel
Thirty Fourth Street EAST at Park Avenue
New York

HILL-TOP-INN
NEWPORT. RHODE ISLAND

May 25, 1921.

Dear Dr. Marafioti:

I accept the dedication of your book with pleasure and pride. Through your researches you have disclosed things about the human voice which restore, in scientific form, the fundamental principles of natural singing, thus giving an inestimable contribution to the musical world.

I, myself, have always felt that something natural has inspired and guided my art. Therefore, since I share your impressions, let me congratulate you and wish you the full attainment of your noble aims for the benefit of future students of the art of singing.

Very sincerely yours,

Enrico Caruso

FOREWORD

THIS book had hardly been completed when the sudden death of Enrico Caruso, the greatest singer of our time, and perhaps of all time, plunged the entire world into grief, and silenced forever the most beautiful and phenomenal voice that the world has known.

This work, dedicated to him in the last days of his life, was conceived as the faithful interpretation of his perfect and rare singing.

For over a decade and a half, I had the privilege of associating with the great artist, not only in the capacity of medical adviser but in the intimacy of a wonderful friendship, and his singing was to me a constant guide and inspiration in my investigations of the many problems of the human voice and vocal art.

By closely observing his method of singing, I saw the correct application by the master himself of the natural laws governing the mechanism of voice production, and I had the opportunity, by testing his ideas and principles, of ascertaining that they conformed with those I have developed in the scientific part of this book.

As a modest wreath of admiration and friendship I lay this work on the grave of the great artist.

P. MARIO MARAFIOTI

339 West 70th Street, New York City

March 3d, 1922.

D. APPLETON AND COMPANY,

New York City.

GENTLEMEN:

I have just received the proofs of the book, "The Scientific Culture of the Voice," by Dr. P. Mario Marafioti, which you are about to publish, and I thank you for the courtesy you have shown me in submitting the advance sheets.

Though there is little time left for me to read and analyze in all its details a work of such importance, I shall, however, not deprive myself of the pleasure of sending you my impressions and opinion on the practical value of this treatise.

As a matter of fact, for the last few years, on several occasions, I have encouraged Dr. Marafioti to pursue his conscientious and patient researches in the particular branch of vocal education which is exclusively identified with science. Indeed, I sincerely believe that it belongs to those men of science who have devoted themselves to the study of the natural functions of the vocal organs, trained for an artistic purpose, to solve the so-called mysterious vocal problem, obscured by the ignorance and the charlatanism of incompetent teachers.

As a matter of fact, from my long practice in singing, and from the experiences accumulated during my career of more than forty years, one point has come to my attention (which has been unanimously endorsed by singers of merited fame), namely, that dramatic singing (that is to say, artistic singing) is the result of two distinct categories of studies:

1. The study of the physiological causes of the natural function of the vocal organs, which in certain cases make the function difficult or even impossible. This part of vocal culture constitutes the "Science of the Voice" (La Science de la Voix), and rightly belongs to the scientists and physiologists who have specialized in this branch of medical research, and are equipped to remedy the shortcomings of so delicate a function as that of the vocal organ.

2. The pursuance of the vocal effects, that is, their proper distribution in the musical phrase, the manner of coloring the tones, the art of expressing with musical tones the varied dramatic sentiments: all these studies constitute the "Science of Singing" (La Science du Chant), and rightly belong to the artist singers who, during their long practice in the art, have acquired a sufficient amount of experience to guide the young aspirants to a career which they themselves have honored before.

This is the thesis treated by **Dr. Marafioti** and which I have so often discussed with him; a thesis that, in my opinion, constitutes a real progress in the development of this art, so human and universal: THE ART OF SINGING.

Believe me, gentlemen,

Yours faithfully,

CONTENTS

xvi CONTENTS

CHAPTER · PAGE

XVI. Caruso's Method of Singing as Explained by Himself 155

XVII. The Radical Reform of Voice Culture Through the Speaking Voice . . . 162

XVIII. The Voice in Its Relationship to Music; the Importance of the Speaking Voice in Voice Culture 186

XIX. The Culture of the Speaking Voice as the Natural Ground for the Culture of the Singing Voice 192

XX. Who Should Teach Voice Culture and How 218

XXI. The Italian Vowels and Consonants as Fundamental Phonetic Elements for Voice Culture 231

XXII. The Articulation of the Italian Consonants; Speaking Exercises for a Correct Voice Production 249

XXIII. Singing Method of the Scientific Culture of Voice; Fundamental Rules for Correct Voice Production 262

XXIV. Vocal Exercises of the Scientific Culture of Voice 278

Conclusion. A Word from a Laryngologist to Singers 303

ILLUSTRATIONS

CARUSO'S METHOD OF SINGING WAS
NOT AN INDIVIDUAL SECRET WHICH
HE ALONE POSSESSED, OR WHICH
WITH HIM CEASED TO BE; IT WAS
THE MOST GLORIOUS EXAMPLE OF
NATURAL SINGING WHiCH WILL REMAIN
FIXED UNTIL NATURE EXISTS NO MORE.

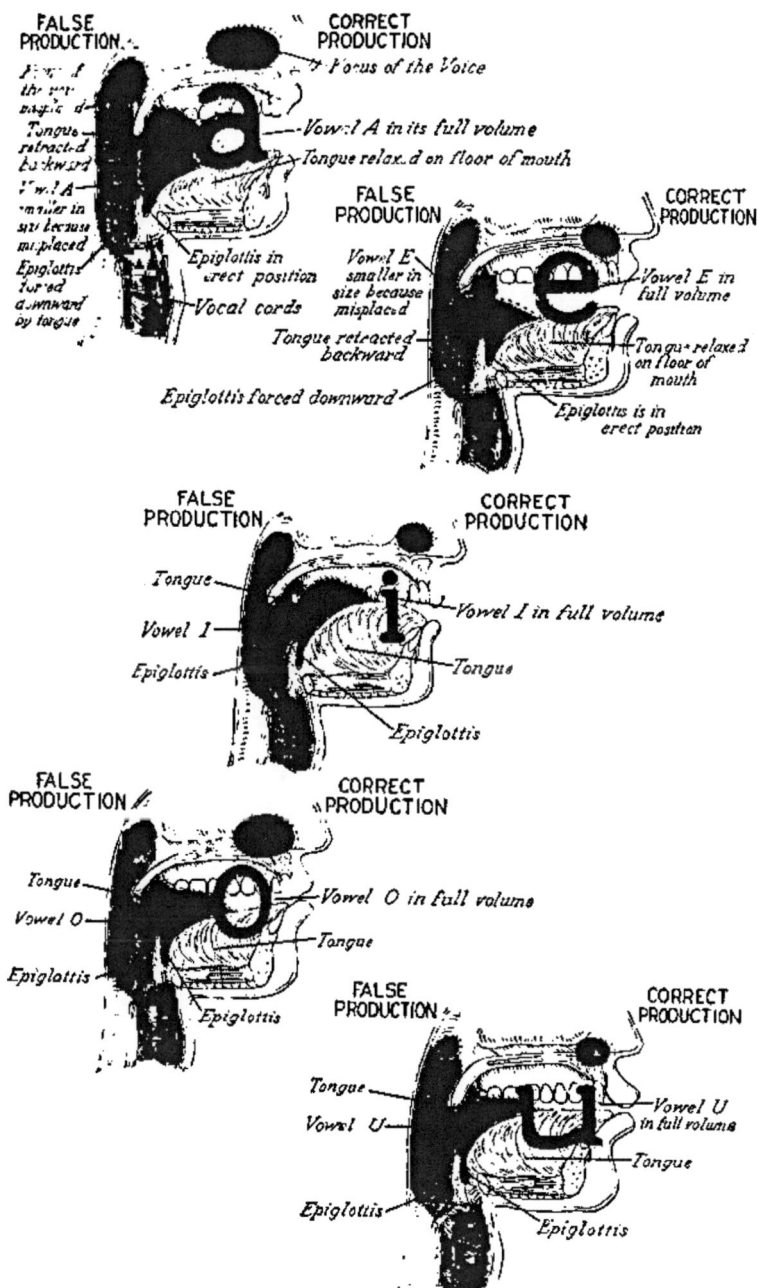

FALSE PRODUCTION

Focus of the voice
the perception of
Tongue retracted backward
Vowel A smaller in size because misplaced
Epiglottis forced downward by tongue

CORRECT PRODUCTION

Focus of the Voice
Vowel A in its full volume
Tongue relaxed on floor of mouth
Epiglottis in erect position
Vocal cords

FALSE PRODUCTION

Vowel E smaller in size because misplaced
Tongue retracted backward
Epiglottis forced downward

CORRECT PRODUCTION

Vowel E in full volume
Tongue relaxed on floor of mouth
Epiglottis is in erect position

FALSE PRODUCTION

Tongue
Vowel I
Epiglottis

CORRECT PRODUCTION

Vowel I in full volume
Tongue
Epiglottis

FALSE PRODUCTION

Tongue
Vowel O
Epiglottis

CORRECT PRODUCTION

Vowel O in full volume
Tongue
Epiglottis

FALSE PRODUCTION

Tongue
Vowel U
Epiglottis

CORRECT PRODUCTION

Vowel U in full volume
Tongue
Epiglottis

FIG. 19— CORRECT AND INCORRECT PRODUCTION OF THE FIVE VOWELS

a. The AIR in the LUNGS which through the

b. SMALL BRONCHIAL TUBES and the

c. LARGE BRONCHIAL TUBES and the

d. TRACHEA is propelled to the

e. LARYNX, putting the vocal cords in vibration and originating *SOUND*.

f. The LARYNGEAL SOUNDS which going through the

g. PHARYNX behind the

h. EPIGLOTTIS reach the

m. MOUTH and are transformed into *VOICE*.

o. The FOCUS or CENTER OF RESONANCE of the voice.

l. The TONGUE relaxed on the floor of the mouth.

n. The UVULA.

k. The opening of the EUSTACHIAN TUBE.

pp. The LIPS, the megaphone of the voice.

rrr. The head, chest and abdominal RESONATING CAVITIES where the vocal vibrations get the resonance of the body.

s. The FRONTAL SINUSES.

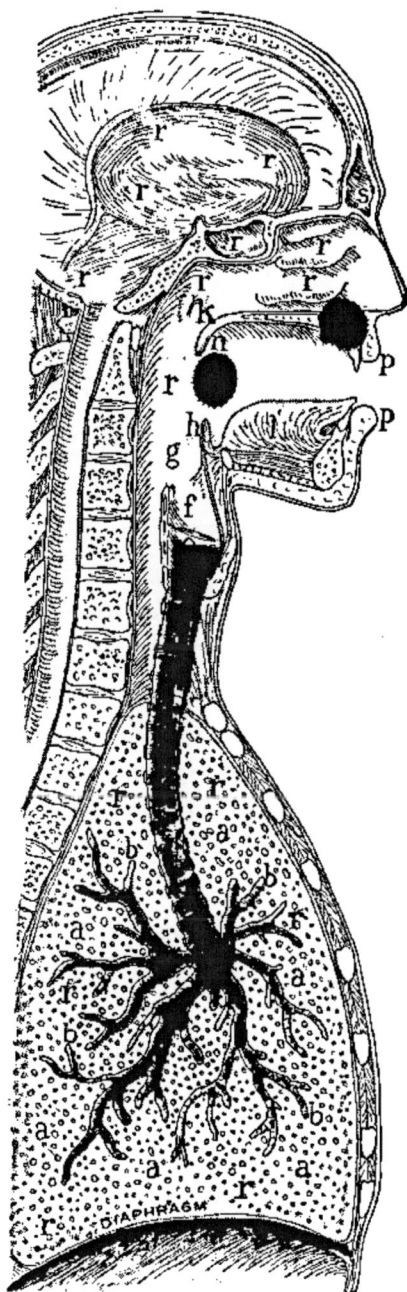

The DIAPHRAGM is shown at the base of the lungs.

THE MECHANISM OF VOICE PRODUCTION CONDENSED IN ONE ILLUSTRATION

CARUSO'S METHOD OF VOICE PRODUCTION

CHAPTER I

ENRICO CARUSO, THE MASTER OF NATURAL SINGING

On February 26, 1873, the most magnificent exponent of the vocal art the human race ever possessed—Enrico Caruso—came into this world. On August 2, 1921, at the height of his glory, his golden voice was stilled forever; and the world, in its grief, is still wondering what it was that Nature bestowed on this privileged son to make him the most wonderful source of human melody of all ages.

Scientists and voice experts vie with each other in trying to explain the vocal phenomenon—Caruso—and, though they differ in their conjectures, they all agree that a voice of such rare beauty, and singing of such effectiveness have never been paralleled in the history of vocal art.

In their various versions, scientists endeavored to trace the striking factors of his rare singing to certain peculiarities of his vocal apparatus, giving most of the credit for his wondrous voice to his vocal

1

cords. This conception, however, merely follows an impression dominating the musical world which has always associated the miracle of Caruso's voice with some secret magic power of his golden throat.

Other experts on voice believe that the principal feature of Caruso's singing was the striking power of his breath, due to the exceptional strength of his diaphragm and intercostal muscles.

A brief analysis can easily prove that the real reasons for Caruso's marvelous singing are not precisely those which have been advanced. He was an exception, not for the rarity of his vocal organs, but for their perfect function—faultless according to natural laws—which made him the truest exponent of natural singing.

Singers endowed with the same and even better vocal organs, on the whole, than Caruso are not scarce, some of them having come under the personal observation of the author. Singers with more remarkable breath-power than Caruso have also existed and still exist. (Tamagno is as yet in the memory of the present generation, without mentioning other living singers.) Yet it is the universal impression that none of them can stand comparison with Caruso as singers.

The truth is that Caruso had nothing exceptional in his laryngeal apparatus, and the larger size of his vocal cords or other peculiarities which have been mentioned about his vocal organs were certainly not the decisive elements in his phenomenal singing. On the contrary, there were shortcomings in his throat which were so evident that if he had had to rely on his vocal organs alone for his career, he would perhaps never have become a singer at all.

As a matter of fact, Caruso himself often commented on this, relating an early experience of his. At the age of twenty he went to one of the most famous laryngologists in Italy, Professor Ferdinando Massei, of the University of Naples, to be treated for tonsilitis at the hospital of Gesù e Maria. When asked about his profession, Caruso said that he was studying singing. The famous physician shook his head dubiously and replied: "Take up something else, you have not the throat for singing."

All laryngologists who had the opportunity of treating Caruso know also that his throat was often much congested, and that he smoked too much, although the beauty of his voice was never impaired.

Therefore his throat was not the magic organ that gave rise to his greatness. This strengthens our theory that the importance given to the throat as the organ which characterizes exceptional voices is greatly exaggerated.

What, then, were the really striking features responsible for Caruso's singing?

My intimate association with the great tenor afforded the opportunity of examining constantly all facts relating to his voice, and the advantage of discussing my impressions with him, accurately studying his own point of view. I, therefore, feel justified in expressing an opinion on this subject, founded on close observation.

Not one, but several, qualifications, physiological

as well as psychological, harmoniously combined in one individual, were responsible for making Caruso the most magnificent vocal phenomenon of the human race. These qualifications are embodied in the words *Natural Singing*.

His vocal organs, most obedient to Nature's dictates, were not anatomically exceptional, but in their physiological function were the most balanced vocal machinery ever known to me. His vocal cords, rather large and thick for a tenor, although not the exceptional factor in the beauty of his voice, gave him the range of a basso as well as tenor. But this is not unusual, as tenor, baritone and basso ranges are conventional, not scientific, divisions. Nature creates voices, the specific qualities and ranges of which have no such scholastic limitations. · Cases of bassos singing as tenors, and contraltos singing coloratura are not infrequent among singers who produce their voices properly. Caruso had one of these rare voices, which he used according to Nature's dictates; thus it was not difficult for him to sing baritone as well as tenor, if he chose to do so. This, therefore, was not the striking feature of his exceptional power. There have been other tenors who could do the same, such as the famous Lablache, who used to sing basso as well as tenor rôles.

One peculiarity worth mentioning, however, about his vocal cords was their rather soft consistency, a circumstance which accounted partially for the mellow and velvety quality of his voice. The value of this is easily illustrated when compared to the marked difference in tone existing between an E string of a violin made of steel and another made of gut, the latter having considerably more mellowness of tone due to its softer consistency.

In reference to the other physical factor commonly conceded as most prominent in connection with exceptional voices, namely, the breath, Caruso certainly always had at his disposal the most generous supply of air, which he supported wonderfully by his control of the diaphragm, that was as strong as any muscle of his body. His beautiful singing, however, was not the result of breath-power, or brute force, but rather of his careful and intelligent distribution of it, which was a remarkable feature in Caruso's style of singing. He always employed only the exact amount of breath required for producing each tone, and no more; and this was responsible for his precise intonation, his remarkable legato, and his long-sustained tones.

Caruso almost unconsciously focused his voice in its most exact pitch, guided by his natural instinct of giving to each note only as many vibrations as were scientifically required. Thus his voice, contrary to the style of singing predominating to-day, was never under high pressure, and, therefore, never sharp.

The natural placement of his voice in the very center of the masque was a most striking feature. Its production was always based on the fundamental tones of the voice, not on the overtones. He used the overtones generously, but only for enriching the fundamental tones, not for overshadowing them.

Generally when voices are forced, the overtones become more prominent than the fundamental tones, resulting in singing which is similar to a painting in which the shadows predominate over the lines of the drawing, making the design indistinguishable. In the singing of Caruso the fundamental design of the voice was clear, solid, and imposing, and its many delicate shadows were responsible for its rare beauty, blending in velvety softness the masculine strength of his baritone quality.

But the exceptional physiological attributes which Caruso possessed were the majestic freedom of his voice production and the striking power of resonance of his body, which he utilized to full advantage. The former was due to his use of the vocal organs in perfect accord with physiological laws, his voice production being so correct, and at the same time so natural, that for the most part singing was for him merely talking. The massive volume and the rare quality of his voice—its exceptional characteristics—were due to the resonance of the body, which was like that of a Stradivarius violin. The much-emphasized properties of his vocal cords, when compared to the striking feature of the resonance of his body, had no more value than the string of a Stradivarius when placed on an ordinary violin. The marked inferiority of tone of the second violin is equivalent to the difference that the vocal cords of Caruso would produce in the throat of another tenor.

Therefore the magic power of his voice lay in the correct physiological mechanism of his voice production, on one hand, and in the remarkable physical conformation of his body, on the other, made up of tissues of exceptional resonant property, acting as an immense resonating case for his tones.

His masque, chest, and all the cavities of his body, even in their remotest corners, were producing sounding vibrations during the correct, free, and expansive production of his voice.

His tongue, of remarkable flexibility, which he could shape in any way, or keep relaxed in a concave form on the floor of the mouth, thereby creating, with his well-arched palate, a larger and rounder space, added not a little to the resonance of his singing.

His nose and frontal sinuses, markedly developed, together with his broad and rounded chest, were striking factors of resonance also. His entire body, in fact, in its large and solid frame, was a striking resonator for his voice.

Therefore all these qualifications, magnificently combined and answering perfectly to the laws of physiology and acoustics, made him the most wonderful exponent of natural singing.

The psychological endowments which lent to Caruso's voice its intense pathos, never before equaled, were supported by the self-assurance of the correct mechanism of his voice production which

gave him the advantage also of devoting all care
to the details of his singing, and to the aesthetic
beauty of his voice molded on its natural sentiment.

For him singing was a pleasure rather than a
technical struggle for effects, therefore, audiences
cried along with him or loved along with him in
his different rôles. His mind, freed from the necessity of thinking high or low tones, was always open
to the inspiration of the words and the music he was
singing. He was the first in his class to abolish
the conventional though beautiful style of singing
of the *bel canto* school, refusing to bend toward the
traditional temptation of making the words slaves
to the tones. He sang the words for themselves—
for their significance—feeling and meaning them.
Hence the pathos of his voice, and his superb enunciation, which made the audience understand and
feel every word he was singing, added much to
his superior standing when compared with other
singers.

Caruso was not a tenor, not a baritone, not a
basso; he was a singer who had the vocal characteristics of all three combined. He had a voice which
did not recognize scholastic, conventional classifications of registers, and ignored all limitations in its
range. He covered all the possibilities of the human
vocal apparatus with the same colorful masculine
voice, from the lowest to the highest tone of his
range. He covered all the possibilities of the human
and at the same time powerful. His voice was a
stream of gold. At the age of forty-eight, when
most singers are at the close of their careers, his

vocal perfection was at its height, and would have lasted however long he lived.

Caruso was a born singer, and a perfect one, by almost divine and superhuman will. He obeyed the call of his heart rather than technical influences, his sentiment being his only guide in singing. Everything in him was instinctive and intuitive. If, at the beginning of his career, he failed to do justice to his vocal gifts, he was unconsciously the victim of technical influences imposed on him by his teachers. His imperfections were due more to psychological conditions than to the voice itself. Surely, though, he did not fail to give the impression that his voice was of rare beauty. When Nature, the real master of his voice, took the lead in his vocal career, and his mind and soul coöperated efficiently, he no longer encountered obstacles in his singing. His evolution as a singer and artist shows very clearly how only lack of artistic education and confidence had held back the natural element which was as powerful in him at the beginning as later.

This very element, though—the natural gift for song—existed and still exists in many other singers, perhaps, as well as in Caruso, but his strong ambition, love of hard work, and intense desire to learn and improve are very seldom combined so conspicuously in one person.

Thus, though Nature endowed him with the rare gift of a most beautiful voice, he owed to himself alone the greater share of his extraordinary success as a singer and artist.

The age of the famous motto of Rossini, that singing requires only "voice, voice, and voice," is gone forever. This was perhaps applicable to the music of his epoch. To-day, to meet the modern psychology and progress, other qualifications are necessary—those which made Caruso the wonder singer of our time.

CHAPTER II

To the making of books there is no end, but the flooding of the musical world with countless publications on the phenomenon of *Voice* makes it imperative for the author to justify this addition to the already voluminous literature on this subject.

The vast majority of the books written in various languages in the last thirty years have, in truth, added practically nothing new, nor influenced to any great degree the development and progress of the art of singing. On the contrary, some of them, by displaying absurd theories based on misinterpreted physiological laws, have caused much damage; and others by simply repeating, in more or less varied forms the principles laid down by such authorities as Tosi, Mancini, Porpora, Garcia, Guillemin, Mandl and Mackenzie have not taken into consideration that those principles can hardly be of benefit to the critical conditions of the singing of to-day, for the art of song has deteriorated very much in recent years, while operatic music has undergone a radical evolution toward interpretation.

An old motto says: "For extreme evils, extreme remedies." The author, therefore, much concerned

11

about the present situation, feels that the time has come to urge a radical reform in voice education. This reform must be founded on scientific laws, and must direct the art of singing toward a fundamental reconstruction better suited to the exigencies of our times, freeing the field of singing from both the unprogressive and empirical, though correct, method of the old Italian school, on the one hand, and the devastating influence of the *arbitrary methods* of voice culture created by incompetent teachers, on the other. This constitutes the *aim* of this book.

No criticism, however, is leveled at the glorious old Italian school of the *bel canto;* but the operatic music of to-day differs widely from that written generations ago. The operas of Wagner, for instance, cannot be rejected for not following the same structure and style as those of Pergolesi, Glück, Mozart, Donizetti, Bellini, etc.; nor should they be limited to few interpreters only because they are more strenuous and difficult to sing. Voices should be trained to such easy production and correct technic, that the length and the intense style of Wagner's or any other modern composer's operas will not expose the vocal organs to any dangerous strain.

We live in an epoch in which, in *every branch* of human knowledge, there has been *progress* and *evolution* from *empiricism* to *scientific principles* and *definite rules*. Music itself, in its different branches, from composition to the technic of instrumental executions, has changed much and

improved. Only the art of singing is still striving
in its empiric form, ruled either by doubtful traditions or by arbitrary methods of singing, the number of which is as large as their practical value is
small. Certainly, if one substantial and correct
method existed, there should be room for no other.

Whose fault, however, if the art of singing is
not only stagnant, but steadily deteriorating?

Some people lay the responsibility on modern
opera. It is true that modern composers write
more elaborate and complex music for singing than
their predecessors; but nobody, in truth, can blame
them for having, under the inspiration of their
genius, directed their works toward new forms of
art, which require more efficient vocal means.

It is our impression that teachers and singers
alone are to blame, if they are not able to face at
ease the new exigencies, and follow the creative
power of these geniuses in their evolution and
progress.

Now, what can be done to change the present
conditions? The author believes that by laying
down a few new scientific principles on the mechanism of voice production and some suggestions for
a thorough reconstruction of voice culture, he has
brought out some original views which should in-
cite the interest of the singing field in the promo-
tion of a radical reform in the art of singing.

The mechanism of voice production and voice
culture cannot be properly used unless properly
taught; and the teaching must be founded on
physiological truths.

The author is not sanguine regarding the immediate effect of this basic reform which he suggests. It takes a long time for truth to win its way in any field of endeavor; but if the advancement of his views has the effect of stimulating discussion and of creating a mental attitude which will lead to the revision of our preconceived notions and to the discarding of worn-out theories, prejudices and superstitions, his efforts will have served some purpose.

Frequently one hears the much abused remark from teachers, "What do scientists know about voice? It is purely an artistic development, and they have no right to interfere with voice culture and the art of singing. This is the domain of the singing teachers alone." The majority of the public accept this statement without discussion.

Yet it is necessary to remind these people that every art has its origin, to a greater or less degree, in some science. They must know that even behind the creation of a musical composition stands the science of harmony and counterpoint, and the structure of its frame and proportions is purely a scientific construction. Any one who knows a little about Beethoven can see in his creations the most vivid example of what science is to music.

The art of painting is based on the science of drawing; and the imaginative power of a painter in creating a beautiful landscape, or in reproducing the character of a person in a portrait, has its origin in the skill of a hand directed by the functional power of the brain. It is, however, obvious that the functioning power of the brain is better known to the psychologist than to the painter himself, and any disorder related to that function can be detected more readily by the former than by the latter. Therefore, science is always of great assistance to art.

There can be no voice without a functioning vocal apparatus, the physiological activity of which gives origin not only to the voice, but to the correct mechanism of its production, which establishes the scientific foundation of the art of singing.

Now, as no one would dispute that the specialist of heart or brain diseases must be well acquainted with the functions of these organs and the treatment of their disorders, no one should doubt that the laryngologist must have a thorough knowledge of the functions of the vocal organs and their physiological product—the voice—and a firmer grasp on the subject than the untaught layman. So, too, he surely must be more able than anybody else to suggest the proper use of the vocal organs for producing a correct mechanism of singing; and whenever a disorder or deformity in voice production develops, he can find the radical means for restoring them to normal.

Therefore, how ludicrous is the statement that the teaching of voice production belongs only to one whose best asset often is limited to the knowledge of how to run a few scales on the piano, or how to read a score; or to those singers who, having sung in defiance of the laws of nature during a brief career, are forced to give it up for the more lucrative profession of vocal instructor.

The public must begin to discriminate between *voice culture* and *artistic vocal education.* The correct training and developing of the physiological functions of the vocal organs during the process of voice production constitutes voice culture. It comprises a knowledge of the normal function of the lungs, as moving power; of the larynx with the vocal cords, as producing power; and of the mouth, which includes the tongue, palate, lips, and the resonance chambers, as resonating power of the voice. To know the defective, as well as the correct, function of all these organs which control the mechanism of voice production constitutes such an important factor in voice culture, that it must be intrusted to the care of responsible experts of the voice, well acquainted with the physiological rules of the vocal apparatus.

The *vocal education* as related to music, that is, operas, songs, etc., is purely a technical study and an acquisition of vocal musical knowledge, which is alike for all musical instruments. That alone should be intrusted to music instructors, coaches, accompanists and conductors.

In face of the alarming condition of the art of singing at present, the author feels fully justified in expressing his ideas on the important subject of voice and voice culture, regardless of any prejudiced or unfavorable criticism. All earnest music lovers should take this stand, and encourage such efforts.

The problem of the responsibilities for the actually harmful condition of voice culture must be solved, and the responsible elements must be denounced without fear. The reaction which may arise from professionals, who are slaves to prejudice, ignorance, or material interests, is to be expected; but if it is true that good singing is fatally deteriorating, all efforts must be combined to discover the real cause, and what must be done to restore the disappearing art of singing.

CHAPTER III

In the preparation of this work the author had constantly before him the question, *who will read this book?*

As a general proposition it may be stated that books on voice do not appeal to the general reader. They are usually of interest only to the so-called musical world and to the few scientific men known as laryngologists. Those who should be particularly interested in a book of this nature are singers, singing teachers and students of singing.

In regard to singers, it is lamentable, but nevertheless true, that the vast majority do not read books on voice. Having made their "success," and having "arrived" (in some cases, of course, in their own belief only), they consider it superfluous to read anything about voice culture. A robust *ego,* often an essential part of the make-up of these individuals, makes them look with disdain on other people's ideas about singing, and they ignore any new viewpoint regarding the phenomenon of the voice, however important it may be.

Most of these singers strive for the applause of the audience, and only for this. It cannot be denied, though, that the average audience, lacking discrimination, is easily satisfied, most easily enthused and aroused to vociferous applause by artificialities, fireworks, and tricks. Therefore part of the responsibility lies with the audience, as for the vast majority of singers its applause is the verdict of the greatness of their achievement and talent, and satisfies all their ambitions. This class of singers, naturally, representing the purely commercial element of the singing field, will not read this book.

It must be acknowledged, however, that there are exceptions. These are the real artists, individuals with ideals, who must not be confused with the mass, and who are always anxious to learn in spite of their real success.

The real artists, having a higher conception of their art, sing for art's sake and do not prostitute art merely for the sake of applause. Conscious of their mission, they hold the applause of the multitude at its proper value, and constantly strive for finer and better expression in their singing.

To them a new viewpoint about voice is deserving of consideration, and they may find some interest in the author's views.

The Singing Teacher

Bernard Shaw has said: "He who can, does; he who cannot, teaches." This may be aptly applied to a condition of affairs now existing in the vocal world.

Teaching is an art requiring great attainments, and not every one can teach. The teacher must have a fundamental basic knowledge of the physiology of the voice, not from mere hearsay, but from actual study and work. He must know physical principles of acoustics, and must have an elementary anatomical and physiological knowledge of the vocal organs. Then, too, he must be a musician, endowed with an exceptionally fine ear, and keen powers of communication in order to reach the average intelligence of pupils.

Considering all these things, I contend that the teaching of singing is a difficult profession, which few are competent to follow. To those few I submit my thesis, and request their constructive criticism.

There is a large class of singing teachers, however, made up of unscrupulous intruders, whose pernicious influence is of inestimable harm both to the competent teachers and to the inexperienced students. The field of teaching is kept in a degraded and unwholesome condition by the malpractices of these individuals who, disregarding, without investigation, any ideas which might throw light on the difficult problems of voice culture, retard its progress and evolution. Their origin is usually traced to studios where as accompanists they have laid the only foundation for their careers. Some of them do not even belong to the musical field. Daring outsiders of any social strata secure admittance to the musical world through connections with singers or teachers, and with no other title or support than their boldness and audacity, gain a foothold in the free land of voice teaching unmolested, taking advantage of the public ignorance and indifference. In this way they succeed in making themselves conspicuous in the domain of voice culture. The unfortunate result is that they find the road to their misdeeds wide open, while it remains closed to the really earnest and competent professionals, who disdain to lower themselves to undignified competition. From this class of unscrupulous intruders the author expects no recognition.

The Pupils of Singing

Enthusiastic, confident, zealous, anxious to learn, and frequently gifted, these credulous young men and women pay the penalty for the ignorance which generally exists regarding voice culture.

A student of any other branch of art or science is requested, nay, ordered, by those who have his tuition in charge, to read all the available literature on the particular subject taught, in order to become familiar with the viewpoints of the various authorities. It is the function of the teacher then to indicate where the truth lies and where the fallacy.

The average singing teacher, however, is not interested in having his pupils read anything except his own literature, from which it is only possible to deduce what a great personage the teacher is. Students often place implicit faith in the ability of masters who, by flattery and falsehood, maintain a hold on their inexperienced victims, until, disgusted and disheartened, the pupils find out too late that their voices have been ruined.

It is lamentably true, however, that pupils expect everything from their teachers, relying very slightly upon their own efforts and responsibility for their future; but if these conditions prevail, it is precisely because they are ill advised.

Of these young men and women, interested in the *truth,* I ask a respectful hearing.

The art of singing is in a very critical condition. Millions have been spent, and are still being spent, for the education of thousands of beautiful voices. for voices of exceptional material exist to-day as heretofore; but where are the good singers?

Yes, there are still a few of the old school who really shine as rare stars in the firmament of song. But when these artists have passed away, shall we have to be dependent upon the phonographic records for beautiful singing as memories of a glorious past?

This pessimistic view is still, however, tinged with hope. That precious gift, the human voice, which more than any other medium reaches the deeper corners of the human heart, will not be hushed. The renaissance of the art of singing must and will come, as surely as the dawn of to-morrow, if we succeed in forcing open the door for a radical reform in the singing world.

By enforcing the laws of Nature, and applying rules based on scientific principles, thus preventing natural voices from being deformed at the beginning of their training, pupils may be taught to sing correctly, beautifully, and easily. Ease is the *sine qua non* of correct singing, as singing means nothing but expressing in musical form sentiments, such as happiness, sorrow, love, which do not require any physical effort to be expressed. A few words spoken in musical rhythm, with grace, color, and artistic expression, are more effective and convincing than the most vociferous, senseless noises, or rasping gutturals, forcibly and acrobatically produced.

Therefore, singers must sing words for their *meaning*, not for their *tones*. It is more important for them to remember this principle than to rely on the top notes of their voices as their strongest artistic resource. Holding a B-flat finale for an exaggerated length of time, to produce a sensational effect for the sake of the audience's applause, is neither beautiful nor artistic. Art is truth, and truth disdains such vulgar display.

CHAPTER IV

THE DECADENCE OF THE ART OF SINGING AND ITS CAUSES; ITS RESTORATION

THE rapid disappearance of good singers has become so alarming in the last few years, that the complaint so widely expressed by those who are concerned about the future of the art of singing seems more than justified.

The deterioration of the vocal art has affected even the Italian school of *bel canto,* which, judging from its contemporary representatives—with the exception of a few celebrities—shows real evidence of degeneration from the glorious old traditions.

The causes responsible for this decadence are growing so rapidly that a solution of the problems essential to the very life of the art of singing has become imperative.

There is no doubt that this critical status of affairs can be faced and successfully overcome, so that the art of song may be restored to its original splendor; but in reality it is a difficult task to carry out such a program, under present conditions.

The downfall of *bel canto* is the result of various and complex causes; the aim to restore it, in view of the present conditions of the teaching field in general, will be severely handicapped, for reasons connected with the commercial element which predominates it at present.

If, however, recovery from the present unhealthy conditions is really desired, it can be attained by radical intervention at the very roots of the pernicious growth—the teaching—a difficult task for any one person to undertake, unless strongly supported by the coöperation of all those interested in the future of the culture of voice.

In a search for the remote causes which brought about the decadence of *bel canto,* most of them can be traced to two primary sources: one musical and the other professional in origin. The first is related to the evolution of singing music, on the whole, and especially of opera; the second to the degeneration of the artistic aims of the modern singers, whose careers have become essentially commercial, and who have forsaken all ideals, to pursue solely a financial and ephemeral success, regardless of how it is obtained. Unfortunately this class of singers furnish the vast majority of the teachers of to-day.

In reference to the evolution of singing music, it must be admitted that the opera has undergone a radical change from its former traditions and style.

Within the last half century a new sense of life, more intense and deep, has opened up new horizons for the display of human emotions in all arts, affecting music most decidedly. The different sentiments which have started to pulsate in the human heart have fundamentally changed the psychology of the world, giving rise to new ideas and feelings, much stronger, more dramatic, more com-

plex—above all—more realistic. In fact, we now
live in an age in which there is no longer room for
romantic sentimentalism, and the ingenuous pro-
ductions which the preceding generations enjoyed
in opera or drama have no longer the power of
interesting the majority of modern audiences.

Therefore, this sudden and radical evolution
which has influenced our psychology—for reasons
and through circumstances which cannot be discussed here—has been transfused and absorbed, in
a natural process of assimilation, by all the different forms and expressions of human sentiment,
through literature, music, painting, sculpture, perhaps principally through the theatrical and operatic
works of recent times.

By natural laws every expression of life must
be subject to the evolution and changes of human
thoughts and emotions; consequently, it is not surprising that these new influences have changed, in
a radical form, the operatic world, its aims, produc-
tions, style, meanings, and the taste of the public
also. Audiences of the last thirty years were getting weary of listening to the arias and duets of
the romantic period of Rossini, Mozart, Bellini,
Donizetti, and their predecessors. Meanwhile the
field of the operatic composers has become influenced by new waves of emotion, more intense
and much deeper, which are gradually taking a
prominent place, substituting realistic and dramatic
musical expressions for the old, conventional melodies and rhythms.

Wagner, the pioneer genius, pressing hard with

his gigantic evolution, the young Italian composers, heralded by the magic seer of the human heart —Verdi, the French, by Berlioz and Bizet—the sparkling painters of colors and sentiment—started the radical reform of the opera, which began to substitute realistic musical mediums for the conventional melodies of the romantic period.

This change has given birth to the so-called modern *truism* and has had a favorable response from the majority of audiences, exercising a very marked influence in the evolution of the art of singing also.   This influence, however, from the standpoint of the *bel canto* style, has proved decidedly negative, though no blame whatever can be laid on the composers of the new operatic music.

The modern Italian realistic school, whose radical operatic evolution was prepared by Verdi's "Aïda" and "Otello," conquered the field so decidedly and in such a triumphant manner with Mascagni's "Cavalleria Rusticana"—followed later by Leoncavallo's and Puccini's operas—that the conquest of public favor seemed almost a spontaneous and natural outcome.   It did not take long for these musicians to put themselves at the head of the operatic reaction in Italy against the old formulas and conventionalities; and while the preceding composers of the past epoch—Rossini, Donizetti, Bellini, and even Verdi in his first operas —were accustomed to write their works either for certain prima donnas, tenors, or baritones, setting the music to their vocal ability, the modern composers, by discarding these practices, gave a higher standing to their works. They began to create operas solely for the sake of the music, regardless of the vocal technicalities of the singers. This new pursuit, more noble, more artistic and dignified, started a new era in the field of Italian opera.

The same transition took place in France, principally through Bizet's "Carmen," followed later by the operas of Massenet, Charpentier, and others, until Debussy and Dukas introduced operas almost musically spoken, such as "Pelleas and Melisande," and "Ariadne and Barbe Bleue."

This new style of music, which abolishes the artificial virtuosity of the romantic period of opera, has naturally been responsible for the sudden change, and perhaps, to a certain extent, for the decadence of the so-called *bel canto,* with no blame, however, reflected on the composers but rather on the singers.

Originally the Italian school of *bel canto* was merely empirical and vague; imparted from teacher to pupil by direct imitation, without definite rules, except for some suggestions resulting from personal experience. By this method the art of singing was transmitted from one good singer to another, and thus from generation to generation.

On the other hand, the operas suited to the taste of the masses were limited in number, almost alike in style, and of popular interest. It was not difficult, therefore, to pass the traditions of their *bel canto* from one singer to the next, by means of the well-known songs and duets of these operas, especially if the pupils were gifted with intelligence and artistic sense as well as with naturally beautiful voices.

When the operatic evolution, however, initiated by the young composers, commenced to gain a foothold in the musical field, the amateur tenors and prima donnas of all singing studios found themselves suddenly confronted with new exigencies, and, instead of applying to the teachers for assistance, in order to make themselves fit to face these novel conditions, they preferred rather to rely on their own judgment, or to follow the suggestions only of those teachers who were more condescending, though less competent. Refusing to go through further training as it was required, the only thing they thought necessary was to learn from a coach or a pianist to shout the rôles of "Pagliacci," "Cavalleria Rusticana," "Bohême," or "Tosca." Therefore, since this epoch, the traditional and patient studying of six or seven years became merely a myth in Italy.

This period marks the *first intrusion* into the *teaching field* of unsuccessful pianists, orchestra conductors, and coaches, who encouraged the impatient singers in the corruption of the art of singing, and later helped, with their incompetent teaching, to hasten its complete decadence.

The realistic style of the modern operas, setting up a very suggestive and temperamental ground, stimulated the young singers to a new manner of singing, more intense and dramatic, above all, more sensational. Attracted by the emphatic and colorful emotions embodied in the rôles of Radames,

Don José, Turiddu, Rodolfo, and Cavaradossi, or Carmen, Santuzza, Tosca, and Manon, they found that there was so much to be displayed through the impersonation of these intense characters that, to sing them properly, or to exhibit sensational interpretations by screaming them, mattered very little in the pursuit of their personal success.

The audiences, in fact, who are usually enthused by anything sensational, gave the stamp of an enthusiastic approval to these first steps toward artistic degeneration. Therefore, a logical reason was no longer seen, nor an actual need felt, for dedicating seven or eight years to the study of correct voice production and artistic singing, as singers of previous generations had been accustomed to do when, in order to sing "Don Juan" or the "Barber of Seville," or "Norma," or "Lucia," etc., a thorough technic and a complete ease of voice production and artistic style had been required.

At the ages of twenty or twenty-one these self-made singers proclaimed themselves the legitimate interpreters of the operas of Mascagni, Puccini, Massenet, Leoncavallo, etc., on the sole support of their natural assets—a beautiful voice and an explosive temperament. The result was soon evident. They entered the operatic field with rare and fresh vocal equipment, and the youthful enthusiasm which such rôles can inspire, but with inadequate preparation. Like young horses whose instinctive enthusiasm for running is uncontrollable, they started their race. A few years of a more or less conspicuous career spent in lavish wasteful-

ness of their natural gift by screaming sensationally
the rôles of Santuzza, Canio, Rodolfo, Mimi,
Tosca, or Butterfly, established the new standard
of the artistic career for these premature singers.
Their creed was summed up in the narrow belief
that in being able to sing the few popular modern
operas, their success was assured, and their ambition was centered only on the applause of the
audience for their high notes, as a means of making
money quickly at any sacrifice.   Art, its noble
mission, its elevating influence, the supreme satis-
faction it gives to its apostles, was completely
ignored or disregarded by this class of singers.
Some exceptions existed, but they were the _rare
aves_ who unfortunately have almost disappeared
at present.

After four or five years these great tenors or
prima donnas, realizing the finish of their hectic
and brief careers, were compelled to seek in the
teaching field the only means for earning a liveli-
hood.   Thus they became the celebrated teachers
of Milan, Paris, New York, London, bringing into
the teaching field, along with their ignorance and
incompetence, the robust egotism which usually
characterizes unsuccessful singers.

From these international centers of art, the
poisonous theories which rule the schools of singing of to-day were spread all over the world,
exercising their disastrous influence on the young
generation of singers.   The Canios and Santuzzas
who had lost their beautiful voices by screaming
like street venders, posed in the musical world as

celebrated teachers. Thanks to an elaborate campaign of publicity they appointed themselves purveyors of the secrets of Italian *bel canto,* and the delicate mission of educating the inexperienced pupils endowed with beautiful voices was blindly intrusted to them.

These pupils formed the second generation of bad singers, and later on, in their turn, became the second and larger set of bad teachers. Certainly what militates in their defense is the fact that they found the field of singing already corrupted at the commencement of their studies, and they had to accept the erroneous doctrines of self-made teachers, who were the ones really guilty of starting the decadence of the art of singing. The responsibility, therefore, for the downfall of the traditional and glorious school must be ascribed to those incompetent teachers who, under the false pretense of being the legitimate representatives of the Italian *bel canto,* spread all sorts of improvised and arbitrary methods of singing throughout the world.

On the other hand, the influence over voice culture exerted by German theories within the last forty years, since the advent of Wagnerian operas, marks another obstacle to the original methods of correct singing.

I do not believe that originally a real German school of singing existed; but if one did exist it was molded on the cast of the Italian school *bel canto.* As a matter of fact, around the early part of the eighteenth century, Giovanni Battista Mancini (born at Ascoli, Italy, 1716) was professor of singing at the Imperial Court of Vienna, where he died in 1800.

It is otherwise known that until some time ago German operas were written on librettos in the Italian language, which suggests the idea that most of the singing teachers were Italians, or had studied the *bel canto* method in Italy.

Before the advent of Wagner, German composers like Händel, Glück, Mozart, Beethoven, etc., were writing their operatic music after the style of the primitive Italian operas. Even the first operas of Wagner were influenced by the Italian school; but later, beginning with Tannhäuser and Lohengrin, the outcome of his newly developed art commenced to gain a foothold in the operatic field, finally establishing the new era of German operatic music with "Tristan," "Meistersinger," and the "Ring."

The transition from Glück, Mozart, and the others to Wagner brought out too decided and blunt a change, so that the soft and delicate modulations of the voice, which most of the German singers had been very particular to develop for singing Glück, Mozart, Bellini, or Donizetti, were no longer sufficient and fit material for the intense, dramatic music of Wagner's rôles. Consequently the deficiency of their vocal means became evident, and created disquietude among singers and teachers. Every one tried to face the new exigencies by using, unfortunately, the instinctive means of compensation for any deficiency, namely, force. They thought that if their voices were not efficient and strong enough for Wagner, there remained but one remedy—to use them to their utmost physical power.

Their conception was indeed erroneous. They did not discriminate between the necessity of training their voices into easier, more obedient and effective mechanisms for surmounting the greater difficulties, but utilized the simpler expedient of forcing their production in order to obtain the required effects. Consequently a few of their number, whose vocal organs were physically very strong and could withstand the strain, accomplished some results by using more power, or, in other words, more breath; the others failed lamentably.

From this class of singers, endowed with exceptional physical resistance, came the German method of singing based on an exaggerated physical efficiency, which was adopted as the only remedy for facing the emergency brought about by Wagnerian music, a method strongly condemned by Wagner himself.[1]

This method, founded on the full power of the breath, supported by the full tension of the diaphragm and other respiratory muscles, was later called by some teachers *physiological*—a false denomination based on a misconception of the real laws of physiology—and which created a false ground for the teaching of voice production in the German schools of singing.

Thus it came about that these erroneous prin-

----

[1] *See* Wagner's *Actors and Singers.*

ciples, based on mechanical force, established the foundations of a method which advanced many erroneous theories about the breathing apparatus and the exaggerated importance of the diaphragm in voice culture. These theories were not confined to the German field of singing alone, but spread all over the world, through the interpreters and teachers of Wagner's operatic music.

The false interpretation of the physiological laws of voice production, started by the Germans, later gave origin to the more elaborate singing methods which are in vogue at present, and to which we owe chiefly the abolition of natural voices, by their incorrect placing and artificial production, based almost wholly on the rules of the chest and diaphragm power.

From these methods of voice culture originated the characteristic type of singer—so popular nowadays—ridiculously conceited, who takes particular delight in asking his admirers to note the expansion of his chest, and test the tension and power of his diaphragm while he is breathing or singing. A wonderful display of brute force, of course, performed by ignorant screamers who feel proud of their athletic achievements, and who never seem to have observed the little nightingale who can sing so beautifully, for hours at a stretch, his voice carrying to great distances, but whose diaphragm is only proportionate to his diminutive size. Evidently the conception of the high-chested singers is that the delicate function of singing is to be compared with the work of a stevedore or a wrestler; and some of the public believe it too, and admire them!

Thus the art of singing, during the period of the operatic evolution, was represented on one side by the temperamental outbursts of the Italian and French singers, and by the athletic and diaphragmatic efficiency of the Germans on the other. Both sides, directed toward a false line of development, not only failed to face the radical evolution of the opera, but hastened the degeneration of the art of singing to the depths that at present are a source of constant distress and anxiety.

Now what is to be done to face this critical situation, and restore the art of singing to a solid and stable basis? Must we go *back* to the old school of *bel canto* and rebuild its method, or must we resort to a *new source,* and establish the foundation of new rules so as to attain a radical reform of the school of singing?

In principle, *progress* is the result of the *incessant evolution* of mankind in its striving for *advancement* and *perfection;* therefore, there is no progress in any branch of science or art in going back a century.

Furthermore, there are several reasons why we cannot revive what has already been worn out in the art of singing of the Italian school of *bel canto.* First, few, even vague rules, if any, have been left by that school which we could set as a standard for the reform we are advocating. Second, its traditional method, transferred from teacher to singer, has gradually been deformed by its adaptation to the vocal equipment of each person, who tried to add to it something of his own individuality and experience; and often, instead of improving the art of singing, brought about the opposite result of contributing to that decadence which in recent years has become so conspicuous throughout.

Third, the exigencies of the school of singing of to-day are very different from those of the past, and therefore must be faced with new equipment, better fitted to the evolution and progress of the present-day music.

Thirty years ago, when a surgeon was called to diagnose a fracture, or a tumor, or to locate a bullet in the human tissues, the only assistance for his diagnosis was the proper valuation of the given symptoms by means of his natural intuition and experience. His professional prominence was then related to his personal skill, and was the only warranty for the importance given to his verdict, though it was not always infallible. Later, the X-ray discovery made it possible for any surgeon to see into the human body and diagnose all surgical cases. Thus the skill itself of the surgeon of thirty years ago no longer has the same valuation, due to the aid of the scientific discovery of the X-ray, and no one to-day would limit a diagnosis to the personal verdict of a surgeon without the confirmation of the X-rays. The surgery of to-day has a real scientific basis.

The great singers of the past, by their natural disposition for singing, by their personal intuition, and by imitation of good examples, were able to achieve perfection in the art of singing. In their older days they were consequently competent singing teachers—celebrities identified with the famous school of *bel canto*. But, like the surgeons of their time, they had no equipment other than their own skill and the painstaking care to follow the intuitive and sole method of teaching of those days, from which they got their own consummate experience.

Would the reviving of that routine in the present condition of the singing field be a possible or self-sufficient solution? By no means. First, because true exponents of the *bel canto* of former times are but memories of the past, and second because the modern repertoire requires much more power and skill, as well as ease of voice production, in order to face the evolution of operatic music. Then, too, another reason—the most important one: the competency of the old masters was in reality not the result of a profoundly conscious knowledge of the art of singing, which could be transmitted in the form of definite and sound principles, but a purely empirical method. These singers of the past, accustomed to sing with the guidance of their ear and the power of imitating their predecessors, were products of both patient mastery and long experience. Their singing was the result of a methodical and gradual training of the vocal organs, with no hasty influence, like the convulsive excitement of to-day. Their method of phrasing aimed more at a perfect production of beautiful tones than at the attainment of psychological expression according to the significance of the words.

Sometimes, in fact, the words of a musical phrase intended to emphasize hatred or contempt were expressed by a most elaborate suavity of tone, merely for the purpose of displaying a beautiful style of singing. The music itself often did not urge much discrimination between different sentiments. A beautiful, inspiring melody sometimes served to overshadow the psychological situation of the opera, creating a conflict of sentiments for the sake of beautiful singing. Certain very celebrated arias, like the famous "Sextette" from "Lucia," for example, show little coherence between the melody and the significance of the words. In some other popular quartets, trios, or duets, the same musical phrases were sung by different singers, all of whom were expressing, in their words, sentiments along different lines, and ofttimes of totally different character, as in the above-mentioned "Sextette" from "Lucia." It was a psychological anachronism of the operatic music which, however, did not vitally affect the indiscriminate and simpler tastes of the audiences of the past.

Yet, from a purely musical standpoint, we do not know if the audiences were in error. It was the period of melody's reign; therefore it was permissible, on the strength of the beauty of the music, to sing with the same purity and sweetness "Spirito gentil" from "Favorita," or "Chi mi frena in tal momento" from "Lucia," regardless of the meaning of the words. But times have changed, and the present epoch witnesses the most radical evolution in the operatic music as well as in the world's psychology and taste. The meaning of the phrase plays the leading rôle in modern music. Human feelings are portrayed in their realistic form, and human voices are intended to express, by the use of singing words, the truth of a dramatic, romantic, or tragic situation, no longer confining themselves to a banal competition with flute or oboe obligato for the mere sake of displaying the flexibility or the purity of vocal tones.

Singers are placed on a more elevated and dignified plane by modern composers, and intrusted with a higher mission by making modern operas less conventional and closer to real human sentiment.

In "Otello," Verdi, though still a devoted apostle of the pure Italian melody because of an elevated sense of art, often refrains from using melodious phrases in situations which call for rapid and realistic developments. The invocation of Desdemona, in fact, "Otello non uccidermi," is expressed by only a few notes of striking effect and conciseness.

Even the commonplace end of "Pagliacci": "La Commedia è finita," or Hanno ammazzato a compare Turiddu" of "Cavalleria Rusticana," have a more effective meaning at that psychological moment than any pompous musical phrases the old-style operas ever possessed.

The new conception of the art of singing as the medium for realistic emotions and situations on the operatic stage makes us look on the school of *bel canto* as an insufficient, time-worn method of singing, just as we look on the conventional construction and orchestration of the old operas, with the accompaniment of the cymbals as old-fashioned works—precious relics of the past, unsuited to our day.

Consequently, the art of singing and the art of vocal culture must be uplifted from its empiric stage, and put on the same progressive and scientific level as all the other arts and sciences. This, and this only, will relieve the present critical situation of the art of singing.

In order then to bring about the radical reform we advocate, we must begin by building up a new method of voice culture on *new foundations,* more modern and concrete, *scientifically correct,* basing it on well-defined *physiological laws.* This will make the method solid, logical, clear, and true enough to be accepted by the vast majority of those who are seriously concerned about the evolution of the school of singing and interested in the future of the vocal art.

We contend that the practical application and evidence of this method has been established by no less an authority than Enrico Caruso, who has so wonderfully demonstrated and reinforced the natural laws of voice production.

His singing, almost faultless, inspired us to investigate the problems of the human voice in its natural production, and gave birth to our conception of voice culture, which claims for Nature alone the right to govern the mechanism of voice production.

The arbitrary methods confined to personal secrets—the creation of singers—and the upbuilding of voices by magic power, should be wiped out as remnants of other ages. One method must be adopted, which should cover all the modern exigencies of voice production and styles of singing, and safeguard very closely the full resources of Nature, priceless in value, as suggested by science, which is infallible. *One method only* for the physiological production of the human voice, as well as for its artistic development and mission.

CHAPTER V

THE following principles regarding the mechanism of voice production, as conceived by the author, were examined by Enrico Caruso during the year preceding his death, and while of much interest to the great singer, were not accepted by him without discrimination. On the contrary, Caruso, attracted by the complex problems concerning the human voice, merely because of his constant craving to investigate and to learn, would not pass over any point without satisfactory discussion, thus becoming the author's most valuable assistant and collaborator in the preparation of this work, both by personal supervision and through correspondence.

During the Summer of 1920, a series of letters were exchanged between the great artist and the author in reference to the contents of this book. It was the author's aim to have Caruso as an adviser and a judge of his work, and while the great tenor showed a decided enthusiasm for it, he was both reserved and inquisitive at the beginning. He accepted, in general, the Principles on the Vocal Mechanism and the suggestions for a radical reform in voice culture as conceived by the author, but for his own conviction he wanted to test them thoroughly.

This desire is plainly expressed in the following quotation from one of his letters, written in a friendly form, and which were not originally intended for publication.

The author now feels that these should be presented in order to justify the title of this book, offering for the reader's examination the actual proof, in Caruso's own handwriting, of how closely the basic principles of the Scientific Culture. of Voice advocated in this book were molded on Caruso's own ideas, and how scrupulous the great artist was before giving them his unconditional approval.

During the month of July, 1920, the author sent to the artist a brief summary of his principles and suggestions for a radical reform in voice culture, which are illustrated in this book. Caruso answered with the following note, the original of which (written in Italian) is reproduced herewith, and which, literally translated, reads as follows:

East Hampton, L. I.
July 22, 1920

DEAR MARAFIOTI:

I am still running after you on Fifth Avenue . . . with the object of discussing what you wrote me yesterday about your vocal principles. What you tell me in your letter is beautiful and convincing, but you understand very well that if Saint Thomas was allowed to *put his finger* you must permit me also to see with my own eyes and thus ascertain for myself your convincing theories. Therefore I will be in New York soon and will come to see you and discuss all this. . . .

Affectionately,
ENRICO CARUSO

FACSIMILE OF CARUSO'S LETTER DATED JULY 22, 1920

Evidently Caruso felt that certain new ideas needed practical demonstration, and only after having made personal observation of some apparatus which the author invented for actual evidence of his principles did he feel reassured in his impressions by this final and decisive proof.

A month later the author sent to Caruso the introduction and part of the scientific section of this book. The following was Caruso's answer (the original, in Italian, of this letter is also shown herewith) :

East Hampton, L. I.
August 23, 1920

DEAR MARAFIOTI:

I am answering immediately your letter of yesterday, as I see I have neglected to inform you that I have read the introduction to your book and find it most interesting. Such an introduction will cause a commotion in the field of vocal teaching, and especially among those who are the merchants of teaching. Among the real professionals I am sure your book will create a deep impression, and will be of major use to them, because, as I see, you add to the teaching of singing also the physical and scientific issues. . . ,

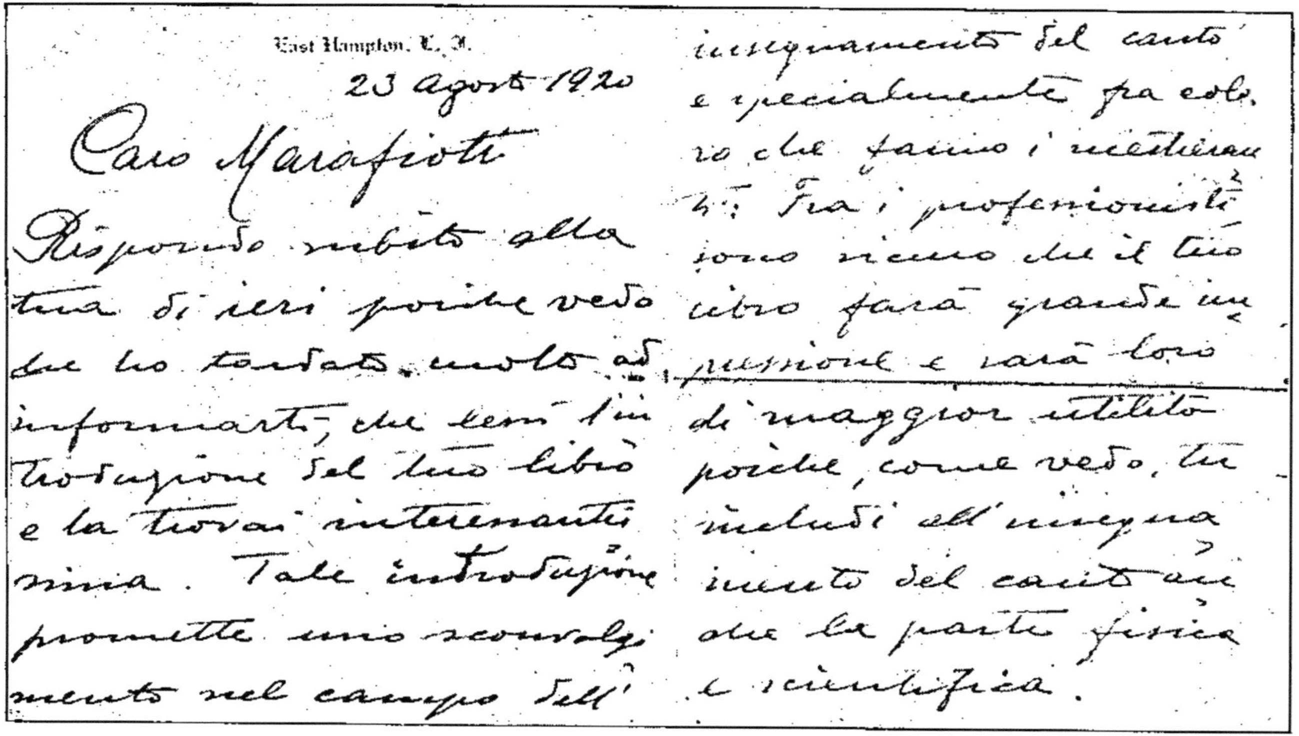
East Hampton, L. I.

23 Agosto 1920

Caro Marafioti

Rispondo subito alla
tua di ieri poichè vedo
che ho tardato molto ad
informarti, che lessi l'introduzione del tuo libro
e la trovai interessantis-
sima. Tale introduzione
promette uno sconvolgi-
mento nel campo dell'
insegnamento del canto
e specialmente fra colo-
ro che fanno i ricettari-
ti. Fra i professionisti
sono sicuro che il tuo
libro farà grande im-
pressione e sarà loro
di maggior utilità
poichè, come vedo, tu
includi nell'insegna-
mento del canto anche
la parte fisica
e scientifica.

FACSIMILE OF CARUSO'S LETTER DATED AUG. 23, 1920

On October 5th the author received the following official endorsement from Caruso for his method of singing—*The Scientific Culture of Voice*

Se gli esperti dell'arte del canto conoscessero le basi sulle quali è fondato il metodo di cultura della voce del Dr. P. M. Marafioti, sono sicuro non ricorrerebbero ad alcun altro metodo.

I principii in esso esposti sono scientifici ma semplici, e si riportano alla sorgente vera della voce, la natura, perciò sono i più corretti.

Gli studenti e le scuole di canto dovrebbero esperimentare questa nuova forma di cultura scientifica della voce, perchè è basata sulle leggi naturali, che regolano il meccanismo di essa, note al Dr. Marafioti come specialista della gola; ed ha un indirizzo moderno rispondente alle nuove esigenze della musica di canto d'oggidì.

Sono lieto di esprimere questo mio personale convincimento, perchè è conforme alla mia stessa concezione del canto; ed il riconoscere il valore del metodo del Dr. Marafioti è semplice giustizia, perchè esso può essere di grande utilità a chi si avvia allo studio del canto ed a chi si trova già nella carriera artistica. Enrico Caruso

FACSIMILE OF ENRICO CARUSO'S ENDORSEMENT OF THIS WORK

which, translated, reads as follows:[1]

October, 1920

If the experts of the art of singing knew the basis on which Dr. P. M. Marafioti's method of voice culture is founded, I am sure they would not resort to any other method.

The principles it sets forth are scientific but simple, and revert to the real source of the voice, Nature; therefore they are the most correct.

Students and schools of singing ought to experiment with this new form of scientific culture of the voice, because it is based on the natural laws which rule its mechanism, known to Dr. Marafioti as a specialist of the throat; and it has a modern tendency, better fitted to the new exigencies of the singing music of to-day.

I am glad to express this personal conviction of mine, for it harmonizes with my own conception of singing; and the recognition of the value of Dr. Marafioti's method is but just, because it can be of great service to those starting out in the study of singing as well as to those who have already entered into an artistic career.

ENRICO CARUSO

During the month of May, 1921, the author read to Caruso a great part of this book, and stated his desire to dedicate it to him.

Three days before Caruso sailed for Italy, he wrote to the author the letter published at the beginning of this book, in which he accepted the dedication and emphasized the point that, since he shared the author's impressions, he wished him the full attainment of his aims.

[1] It should be noted that special care has been taken to make a literal rather than a literary translation of the original.

On the strength of these personal testimonials of Caruso, the author feels justified in his claim that, though the method he is presenting as Caruso's Method of Singing has not been written by the great singer personally, nevertheless it is the most faithful reproduction of his own ideas, and above all, of his "feelings" about his own singing. No singer, especially a great singer who is born such can explain exactly how he sings, though he may express his "feelings" about his singing.

The following principles outline the scientific contents of this book, on which the author bases his *Radical Reform of Voice Education.* Some suggestions will be developed later, indicating how this reform of voice culture can be carried out practically. The principles are:

1. *Voice* is *Speech,* and is produced by the *mouth,* not by the vocal cords. The *vocal cords* produce only *sounds,* which are transformed into *vowels* and *consonants* by a phonetic process taking place in the *mouth,* and giving origin to the *voice.*

2. (*a*) The full extension of the natural range of the voice is produced only by using the *minimum tension* of the vocal cords and the *minimum breath* required for each tone. This establishes a correct mechanism of voice production.

(*b*) The laryngeal sounds must be transmitted to the mouth *free* of any interference; *freedom* is the fundamental pillar of voice production.

3. Breath is an indispensable factor in voice production, but *it is not the essential power* which develops the voice as it is taught to-day. On the

contrary, the function of *singing* develops the *breathing apparatus* and its power, just as any physiological function develops the organ from which it takes origin. Therefore *singing* develops *breathing,* not *breathing,* singing.

4. *Resonance* is the *most important factor* in voice production. It furnishes to the voice volume and quality, and emphasizes its loudness. To rely on resonance rather than on force is essential for producing a big and pleasing voice.

5. *Speaking* and *singing* are *similar functions,* produced by the same physiological mechanism; therefore they are the same vocal phenomenon.

The speaking voice is the substantial factor of the singing voice and singing, in its very essence, is merely speaking in musical rhythm; hence no correct singing can exist without a correctly produced speaking voice.

6. The *pitch* and the *dimensions* of the singing voice—the volume, the quality and loudness—are determined by the *speaking voice.* Speaking high or low, resonant, loud or soft, in any gradation of sentiment and shade of color, lays the ground for singing in high or low pitch, loud, resonant or soft, in any musical color or expression.

7. There are *no registers* in the singing voice, when it is correctly produced. According to natural laws the voice is made up of only *one* register, which constitutes its entire range.

CHAPTER VI

To reinforce the foregoing principles, the author advances the following suggestions which can bring about a radical reform in the culture of the voice, directing the art of singing toward more definite rules, scientific, and better suited to the modern conditions:

1. Voice culture must be *natural* in its basis, and *scientific* in its principles—not *empiric* and *arbitrary*. There must be only *one method* of singing, founded on *physiological laws,* presented in practical form.

2. The *education of the voice* must begin in the *elementary schools,* and must first be taught to children in the form of correct use of the *speaking voice.*

We believe this to be the *most important* feature in the reform of voice culture, being directed to the very origin of what is responsible for the initial defects and deterioration in the natural voices of children. A *school* should be founded for this purpose, where school *teachers* could get adequate instruction in the natural and *correct phonetic rules, molded on classic languages,* for teaching this form of voice education.

3. Singing teachers must be *new professionals*, combining *scientific* with *artistic* knowledge; a class of *voice specialists,* differentiated from coaches, accompanists, vocal musicians, etc.

4. Voice specialists must undergo a regular course of training in scientific and musical matters related to voice, and *must be subject* to *examination by a special Board of Scientific* and *Musical Experts, elected* or *recognized* by the *Government.* They must get their *practicing licenses* from this Board, as in the case of other professions. That alone can protect the singing field from all kinds of intruders, charlatans and impostors.

A survey of these principles and suggestions discloses the *extent of the author's task.* In his endeavor to demonstrate how certain ideas about the mechanism of voice production have been entirely neglected or misinterpreted, and for strict adherence to the principles laid down, which differ considerably from the methods now taught, he *must advocate* and *suggest* an *almost opposite form of vocal education from that which is now in vogue.*

That has no relation of any sort with the completion of the culture of the voice, as far as musicianship, technic and style of singing are concerned. This is a task which belongs to a class of professional people, who represent the musicians of the voice. These professionals—coaches, accompanists, interpreters, etc., have the function of finishing the artistic education of the pupil for the stage or any other career. *But the preliminary voice education of the singing students is quite another matter, to which more serious and solid care should be devoted,* and in which the *untaught should take no part* whatsoever.

For this purpose the author proposes a new form of voice education which he calls the *"Scientific Culture of Voice,"* based, as above stated, upon the fundamental laws of acoustics and physiology of the voice, and molded on the method of singing of Enrico Caruso, who has been the living model of the natural mechanism of voice production. This culture must be intrusted to the specialists of the voice who, being well equipped with the necessary scientific and musical knowledge, fill the requirements for competent and correct teaching.

The contents of this book, therefore, will treat first of the voice purely as a physiological phenomenon, from the standpoint of its natural production, in accordance with the principles already announced, and then of the most effective means for accomplishing a radical reform in voice culture. This will be carried out by an entirely original method, based on phonetic rules molded on the Italian language, which places and develops the singing voice through the speaking voice.

CHAPTER VII

THE human voice is a physiological phenomenon produced by the vocal apparatus.

Two branches of science — Physiology and Acoustics—govern the human voice. Physiology, which rules the functions of the human body, controls the mechanism of voice production; and Acoustics, which treats of the laws and properties of sound, controls the physical product of the vocal apparatus—the sound.

As a fundamental element of the art of singing, however, voice represents a higher and more complex factor than sound, as it constitutes the artistic medium for expressing our thoughts and feelings through music. Therefore, for the full exploitation of the phenomenon—voice—the support of intellectual assistance is required, and that is supplied by Psychology, the science of the study of intellect and sentiment.

Psychology lends to singing its mental contributions—its inspiration, its emotions, its color, its style; all artistic features which do not belong to the voice in its simple form of physical sound.

This psychological contribution constitutes the most precious equipment in the art of singing and can be defined as the *Sense of Singing*. The sense of singing stands to the physical phenomenon of voice as the painter's conception of life and colors—which he carries out through his imagination and feelings—stands to his hand and brush.

We believe that the sense of singing is entirely a natural gift, which no book or teacher can confer upon any pupil to whom Nature has denied it. Education may assist in developing it, but there must be a substrata of certain mental qualities which can be cultivated to make it possible to achieve this fundamental factor of the art of singing.

Therefore, the task of illustrating the contribution of Psychology to this art will not be part of our aim in developing this book. It is too important to be treated briefly, in outline form, and it is of no real value in the preliminary, though most essential, task of teaching the mechanism of voice production. Students of singing, however, must note that psychology constitutes the very soul of the art of singing, and must not neglect the education of their minds, which comes first in the exploitation of every art.

In regard to the physiology of the voice, in spite of all the doctrines and books written about it, there seems to be no clear understanding among professionals of the laws and rules which constitute the foundation of the physiological voice production and culture. Many, in fact, confuse *physiological functions* with *physical efforts,* and their misconception goes to the extent of condemning the real laws ruling the function of singing because they attribute to the term "physiological" the qualification of effort.

In reality *physiological,* when related to a function, is equivalent merely to *normal.* The misunderstanding on this subject is due principally to the fact that the greater part of the singers of our times in producing their voices employ a power which is the result of their maximum energy, and they gauge it as normal, while in reality it is not. As a matter of fact normal efficiency is produced by the minimum of energy. A motor car running at the speed of one hundred miles is not ruled by its normal power, its motor being under high pressure.

The voice produced by the maximum energy of the vocal organs is under a strain, while the minimum of power produces its normal efficiency. This normal efficiency is what should be conceived as the *physiological function.*

The multitudinous theories about breathing, breathing exercises, diaphragm development, voice building and many other complicated suggestions related to the mechanism of the voice, show how incorrect is the knowledge of the functions of the vocal organs and how far these functions are from being performed by physiological mechanism. Voice production in reality is as simple and spontaneous as is any other function of the human organism. That constitutes the wonderful asset of Nature—simplicity.

A clear conception of the function of the vocal apparatus and the mechanism of voice production cannot be attained without, at least, an elementary knowledge of the anatomy of its different organs, and of the fundamental laws of acoustics which rule them. But a thorough anatomical study of the different organs of the vocal apparatus is not really necessary for the comprehension of the principles of voice culture. Such information may be necessary for teachers, but it is as unnecessary for the student to know the different muscles and cartilages of the larynx as it is for the dancer to have a detailed anatomical knoweldge of the muscles of the legs. Too much emphasis has been placed upon the necessity of the study of anatomy for pupils. We believe that the student should know only what the mechanism of the voice is, and what the different organs are that take part in the production of this mechanism. The teacher should acquire a thorough knowledge of the vocal organs, but most essentially of their functions, in order to be able to determine whether the pupil's work is correct, according to physiological rules, or whether it is incorrect because of a faulty mechanism in the voice production.

In the next chapter an outline will be given of those few anatomical parts which are necessary for the study of the voice, omitting all unimportant and complicated data.

Of the other scientific branch, concerned with the phenomenon of the voice—*acoustics*—it is enough to bear in mind a few elementary principles related to the fundamental laws of the sounds.

Sounds are the physical result of bodies in vibration. Vibrations are movements traveling in every direction, which reach our ears and are perceived in the complex form of sounds, if periodic, of equal duration, regular and rapid. If they are irregular and unequal in duration, they are perceived merely as noises.

This difference is very important because it establishes from the very roots of the physical formation of the voice the fact that only *equal vibrations* can produce *perfect sounds* or *tones;* therefore, equal vibrations are the fundamental asset for a *correct form* of *singing.* That makes it very evident how strictly the laws of acoustics are connected with the rules of physiology in the production of the laryngeal sound which is the seed that generates the wonderful phenomenon of the human voice.

Therefore, the correct physiological mechanism of voice production, by generating equal vibrations, establishes the basic foundation for a correct and natural method of singing. It is obvious then that the mechanism of voice production is fundamentally controlled by the laws of both sciences—Physiology and Acoustics—working in harmonious coöperation.

CHAPTER VIII

In giving a brief survey of the anatomy of the vocal apparatus we will avoid as much as possible scientific terms, exhibiting in simple form only what is indispensable for singers to know about the physiological functions of those organs which represent the essential factors of voice production.

The mechanism of the human voice consists of three elements: the moving power, or breathing apparatus; the producing power, or laryngeal apparatus; and the resonating power, or resonating apparatus.

These three elements are organized as follows:

1. The moving power consists of the lungs, the respiratory muscles, the bronchial tubes, and the trachea.

2. The producing power, the larynx, its muscles, cartilages, and vocal cords.

3. The resonating power, the pharynx, the mouth, and the chambers of resonance.

The author includes among the chamber of resonance all the body's cavities.

The *lungs* are two bellows of spongy tissue which contain a large number of little cavities filled with air (the air we inhale). To these cavities are joined numerous small tubes, called bronchial tubes, which run into the lungs carrying the air and becoming gradually larger in size and fewer in number. Toward their exit from the lungs the bronchial tubes

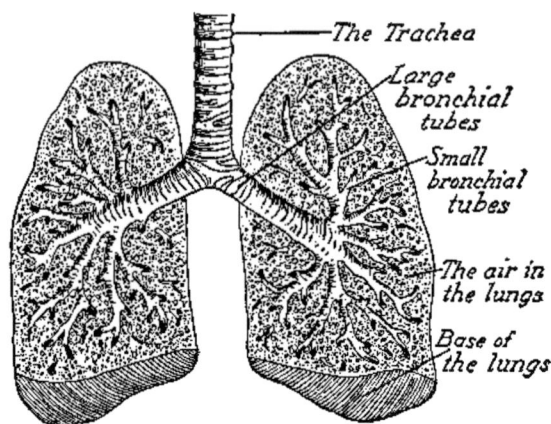

FIG. 1.—THE LUNGS

are reduced to two—the large bronchiae, and finally to one—the trachea (Fig. 1).

In the second figure the lungs are contained in a cage (the chest) which is formed by the ribs and the intercostal muscles, attached between the ribs. Under the lower border of the lungs, adherent to the spinal column and to the lower six ribs, lies a large and strong muscle called the diaphragm. Its function, very important, though very much exaggerated by some improperly called physiological schools of singing, is a coördinate movement of contraction and relaxation, which, in connection with the movement of the other muscles of respiration, establishes the mechanism of breathing by enlarging and reducing the chest and lungs to their normal position.

The *larynx*, the second element of the vocal apparatus, represents the sound box of the vocal

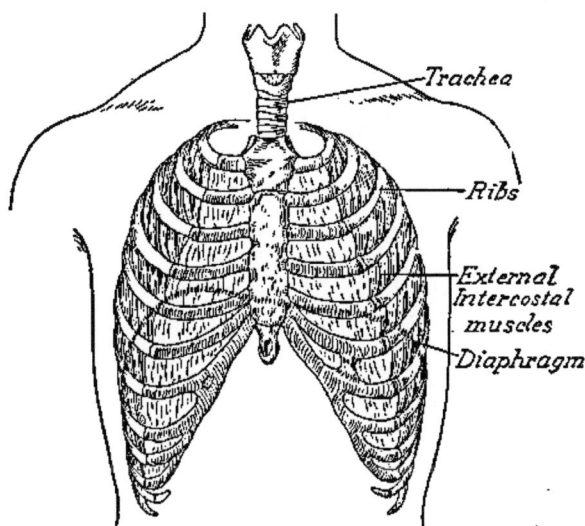

FIG. 2.—THE CHEST

organs (Fig. 3) and embraces its cartilages and muscles, and, most important, the two elastic bands called the vocal cords.

The cartilages of the larynx, situated above the trachea, are the following: the cricoid and thyroid, the arytenoids and epiglottis (Fig. 4), and the two smaller cartilages (Santorini and Wrisberg) which are of minor importance. All of these cartilages are joined by ligaments and muscles, which move the larynx, and adapt the vocal cords to the different adjustments for producing the relative sounds.

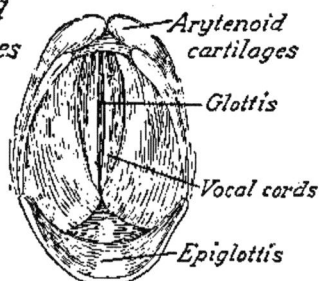

The vocal cords (Fig. 4) are two elastic bands, inside of the larynx, kept in tension during their vibratory function by the cartilages and the muscles, so that they can be put in vibration by the blast of air pushed by the lungs and produce the sound. The fissure between the vocal cords is called the glottis. The vocal cords, in a position of rest, are re-

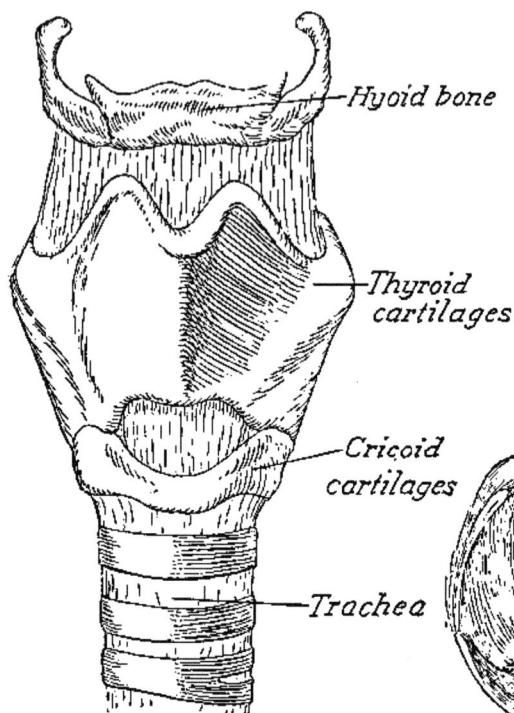

Hyoid bone

Thyroid cartilages

Cricoid cartilages

Trachea

Arytenoid cartilages

Glottis

Vocal cords

Epiglottis

FIG. 3.—THE LARYNX   FIG. 4.—THE VOCAL CORDS

laxed and wide open, thus leaving a larger space for the passage of the air, which is called the glottis.

In the upper part of the larynx there exists a very important cartilage called the epiglottis (Fig. 5). The epiglottis is flexible and is situated between the base of the tongue and the opening of the larynx, Its function is doubly important, since it acts as a protective lid to the glottis, by closing the larynx in swallowing, so that food and drink may pass over it without exposing the breathing apparatus to any danger; and in singing it lends free passage to the sounds, from the vocal c o r d s to the mouth and chambers of r e s o n a n c e, by holding itself in an erect position, so as to leave the larynx wide open. The epiglottis is attached to the b a s e o f t h e tongue and their relationship is very im-

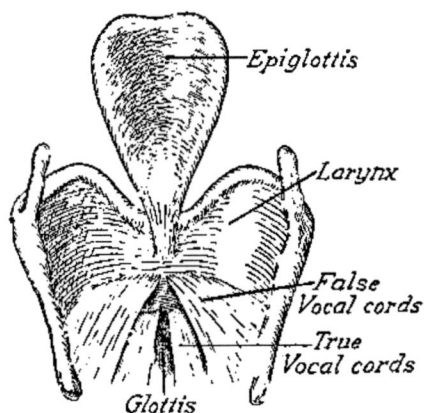

FIG. 5.—THE EPIGLOTTIS

portant, as together they play one of the most essential rôles in the mechanism of voice production, to which, unfortunately, not enough consideration has thus far been given.

The third element, *the resonating power,* consists of the pharynx, the mouth, and the chambers of resonance.

The pharynx (Fig. 6) extends from the opening of the larynx to the opening of the posterior nasal cavities, and includes also the uvula, which represents the boundary between the pharynx and the mouth. The upper part of the pharynx is called the nasopharynx and is an important factor for the resonance of the voice. The uvula is attached to the soft palate and is prominent in the mechanism of the voice, because it has the faculty of controlling the opening and the closing of the posterior nasal fossae. By this func-tion the nasal reso-nance c a n b e im-improved or checked.

T h e mouth (Fig. 7), the very important organ of voice pro-duction, is the cavity w h i c h contains the tongue — the invalu-able factor in speak-

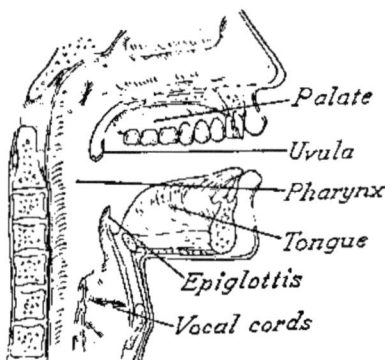

FIG. 6.—THE PHARYNX

ing and singing—the palate, and the lips. Above the palate are the chambers of resonance, which consist of the so-called masque, made up of all the cavities, frontal sinuses, antrum, etc., of the upper

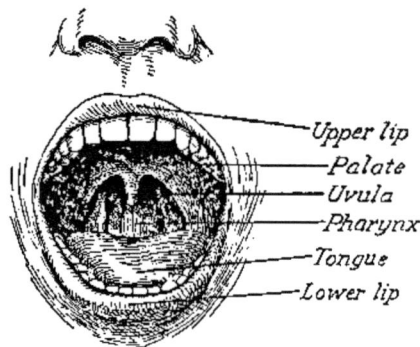

FIG. 7.—THE MOUTH

maxillary and frontal bones.

All of these organs above described are parts of one single apparatus, which is formed by a long tube going from the mouth to the lungs, called the vocal ap-paratus. This ap-paratus has the mission of producing and carrying the breath from the lungs to the vocal cords, which puts them into vibration and produces the sounds. From the vocal cords the sounds are carried, by the breath, to the mouth, where they are transformed into voice, and to the resonance chambers, where they get their full resonance.

The resonating power, however, is not represented by the resonance chambers alone, but by all the cavities of the entire body, according to the author's view, which will be more fully discussed in a later chapter devoted to resonance.

In order to enable the reader to obtain a full view of the entire vocal apparatus, the author has condensed in the accompanying illustration (Fig. 8) all the organs that take part in the formation of the voice. The most important of them are specially indicated.

The illustration is a transverse section of the vocal apparatus. Familiarity with it is of great help in the study of the mechanism of voice production. Therefore we recommend to the reader a thorough examination of it, starting from the bottom and working up. Held by the convexity of the diaphragm are the lungs. From them originate the small bronchial tubes, which gradually become the two large bronchial tubes which, in their exit from the lungs, converge into the trachea. At the top of the trachea is the larynx, which contains the vocal cords. At the opening of the larynx stands the epiglottis, which is attached to the base of the tongue. Then follows the pharynx, the uvula, the mouth, the palate, and the resonance chambers.

The task of demonstrating the important functions of these organs belongs to physiology, which, by means of its natural rules, can give the very

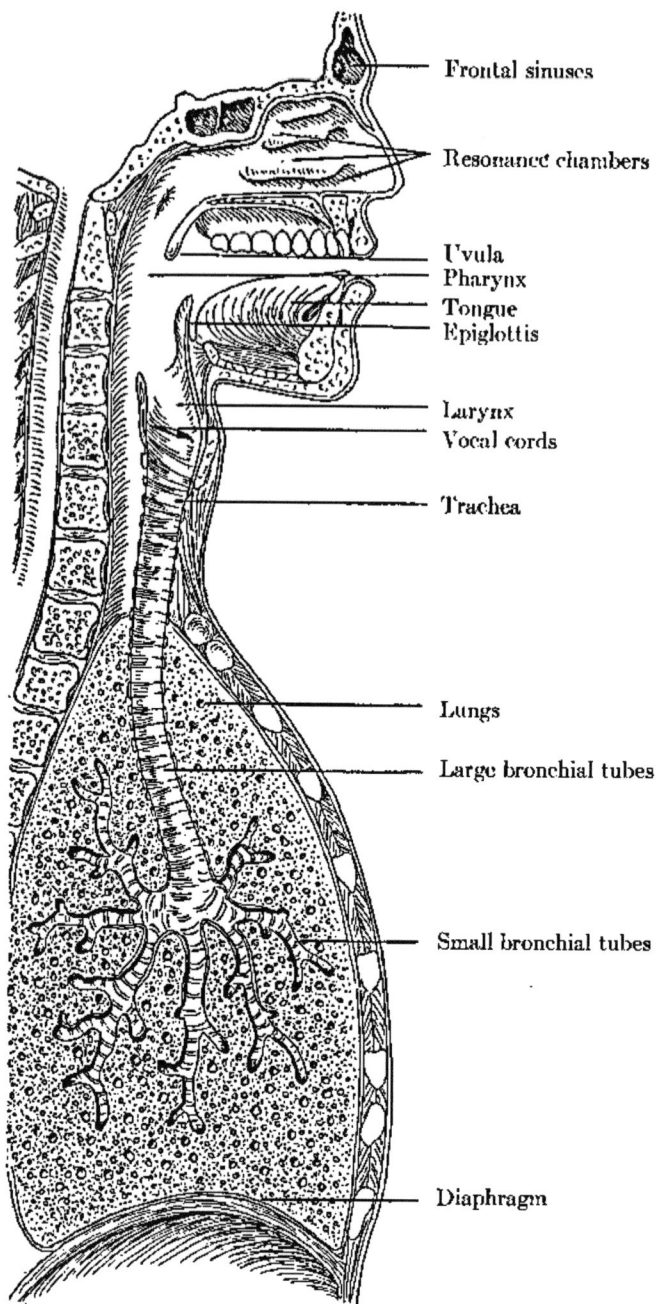

- Frontal sinuses
- Resonance chambers
- Uvula
- Pharynx
- Tongue
- Epiglottis
- Larynx
- Vocal cords
- Trachea
- Lungs
- Large bronchial tubes
- Small bronchial tubes
- Diaphragm

FIG. 8.—TRANSVERSE SECTION OF THE VOCAL APPARATUS

67

correct exhibition of the mechanism of the voice. This preliminary knowledge of the vocal apparatus and of the fundamental laws of acoustics prepares the ground for the development of our principles, in reference to voice production, the aim of which is centered, according to our conception, on closely following the dictates of nature.

CHAPTER IX

VOICE is *speech,* and is produced by the *mouth,* not by the *vocal cords.* The vocal cords produce only *sounds,* which are transformed into *vowels* and *consonants* by a phonetic process taking place in the *mouth,* and giving origin to the *voice.*

It is a general belief that voice is produced by the vibrations of the vocal cords. "A column of air, going from the lungs through the trachea to the larynx, strikes and puts in vibration two ligaments, and produces a sound. The ligaments are the vocal cords, and the sound, produced by the vibrations, is the voice." This is the definition given, in more or less similar form, by the majority of writers on voice.

The author believes that a moment's thought on the subject will show that this definition is not correct, as there is a marked difference between simple sounds, as produced by the vocal cords, and the real phenomenon of Voice.

Going back to the origin of the word Voice, in its root it means *speech* (voc, in old Sanscrit, "to say": Vox, in Latin, "to speak"); and has been associated, since its origin, with the qualification of a sound uttered by the mouth in the form of speech or song. The real essence, therefore, of the physical product of the vocal apparatus—the voice as *speech*—was established since the birth of civilization by means of the old classic languages.

Scientifically sound is the physical product of equal vibrations given by any vibratory matter. When the vibrations are produced by the vocal cords they give origin to the laryngeal sound, musically called *tone*.

Voice is a more complex phenomenon, in the formation of which the sound is essential, but is not the only factor, as for the formation of the phonetic elements of the voice—the vowels and consonants—the coöperation of other organs in addition to the larynx are required.

As a physical phenomenon the vibrations of the vocal cords are nothing exceptional, as they can be produced by any sounding body—a musical instrument as well as the human instrument, the larynx, which in its structure is nothing but a musical box combining the properties of both a wind and string instrument. If two elastic strings which are kept in the same tension as the vocal cords are struck by a blast of air similar to that which can put the vocal bands in vibration, they produce a sound physically similar to that of the vocal cords, but much different from that which characterizes the human voice. This shows that the vocal cords alone produce sound, not voice.

There is no physical difference between a laryngeal sound and a violin sound; but there is a decided difference between the violin sound and the human voice in its real characteristics, as the former has no power to produce phonetic elements—words. This demonstrates that sounds do not possess the physiological properties required for making voice.

Therefore the *laryngeal sound* and the *human voice* are not exactly the same thing, and although sound is the germ from which voice develops, *it is not the voice.* It stands to the voice as the seed to the plant, which is an outgrowth of the seed but is no longer the seed itself.

This implies that the rôle played by the vocal cords in the formation of voice is much overestimated. They are the leading factor in as far as the production of the sounds is concerned; but the formation of the voice is caused by the phonetic apparatus —the mouth. The resonance chambers complete this process of evolution by adding to the voice their resonating power, with all the characteristics attached to it—volume, quality, and loudness.

The voice, therefore, in its complete form, as produced by the mouth, is much bigger, more resonant, and of better quality than the original sound from which it takes its origin. This establishes a marked difference between the two products of the two different phases of voice formation— the laryngeal, which creates the sound—and the phonetic, which creates the voice.

If, however, the principle that the vocal cords produce only sounds and not voice is demonstrated, it consequently becomes evident how erroneous it is to attribute to them a function which they do not perform, at least entirely. The vocal cords in fact are apt to produce perfect tones, though always throaty and rather weak if hindered from getting the full resonance of the resonance chambers; but it is not in their power to produce any kind of voice, composed of phonetic elements, vowels and consonants, without the full coöperation of the mouth—the real center of the voice.

John Hullah, professor of Vocal Music, in Queen's College, London, said: "There is no singing without saying: that which is sung must also be said." This statement—the result of a logical intuition—has great value, regardless of the fact that it is not based on any scientific principle.

The following conclusions, which are of great importance, follow the principle of "that which is sung must be said":

1. Singing, depending on saying, must rely on voice, or words, and not on sounds.

2. The decided difference between sounds and words brings about the result that the former, being produced by the vocal cords, are sung in the larynx; and the latter, being composed of vowels and consonants, produced by the mouth, must be sung by the mouth. This establishes, from the beginning, the physiological rule that the voice must be placed in the mouth.

3. Voice being produced by words, the more perfect their formation, the more perfect is the resulting singing voice. It is evident, then, that the singing voice depends entirely on the speaking voice, which establishes the important rule that *for training the singing voice correctly it is essential, to train first, the speaking voice.*

This fact upholds the irrefutable axiom that any method of singing based on tone and not on voice production, in other words, based on laryngeal production of sounds, is to be condemned, as it tends to the abolishment of the natural beauty of the full voice for the purpose of developing only beautiful sounds, like the sounds of any musical instrument. In such case the tones, being placed in the larynx, are only slightly reinforced by the laryngeal resonance, because they do not expand enough to reach the masque.

A beautiful voice, in truth, must be the result of a simultaneous collaboration of the different organs which constitute the vocal apparatus—the moving, the producing, and the resonating power—and therefore cannot be confined to a laryngeal struggle between the exaggerated efficiency of the moving power (breath) and the strain of the producing power (vocal cords).

Only by the *complete coöperative and harmonious work of these three powers* is it possible to obtain the desired result of producing a *perfect mechanism of singing, ruled by natural laws.*

Great singers' voices, especially natural voices, have always been associated with the belief that something rare exists in the anatomical structure of their vocal apparatus—exceptional vocal cords, for example, different from those of the generality.

The author has had the opportunity (through his professional connection with one of the most prominent operatic institutions in the world) of examining and studying the vocal organs of almost all the greatest singers of the present day. In the majority of them the vocal cords did not present any striking characteristics which could establish a marked difference when compared with the vocal cords of people not gifted with singing voices. On the contrary, among those singers whom he had the opportunity of observing, were some with rather deficient vocal organs, and often affected with chronic congestion of the vocal cords, which, however, did not interfere with their singing. In fact, in a few cases the voices were exceptionally good; Caruso was a typical example of this class.

On the other hand, the author has seen vocal cords of exceptional character in persons who had not the slightest notion that they could sing and develop beautiful voices. The belief, therefore, that the vocal cords of singers are responsible for the power and the beauty of their voices, and are the source of their exceptional singing, is as false as it is popular.

In reference to our conception of the mouth as the physiological center of the voice, illustrated in this chapter, it may be argued that this principle can be accepted only in regard to the speaking voice, but does not apply to the singing voice. According to our idea, however, speaking and singing are similar actions; therefore there is no fundamental difference between the speaking and the singing voice. The reader, in the fifth and the following principles will find this subject illustrated at length, with the refutation of all objections that may arise.

CHAPTER X

1. THE full extension of the natural range of the voice is produced only by using the *minimum tension* of the vocal cords and the *minimum breath* required for each tone. This establishes a correct mechanism of voice production.

2. The laryngeal sounds must be transmitted to the mouth *free* of any interference; *freedom* is the fundamental pillar of voice production.

When the mechanism of voice production enters into action, the breathing apparatus, by means of its respiratory muscles, pushes the air toward the vocal cords and puts them in vibration. The vocal cords, which by a coördinate function of the muscles and cartilages of the larynx come together, because of their elasticity adapt themselves to an indefinite number of adjustments and give origin to a series of different tones which constitute the range of the voice.

The embryonic sound, resulting from the vibrations given by the *minimum* of *tension* of the vocal cords, put in vibration by the *minimum* of *breath*, constitutes the lowest tone of the natural range of the voice as produced by a correct mechanism.

75

This tone is very feeble and is of no practical use in singing, but serves to great advantage in the mechanism of voice production, as it establishes the deepest point of support for the consecutive tones of the range, like the cornerstone in the foundation of a building.

By comparing the upbuild of the natural range of the voice with the construction of a house, we see a great similarity in the structure of both, which tends to show how important is the low section of the vocal range in the production of the voice.

The foundation of a building is the underground section which readily escapes observation; yet it is as important as the section above ground, if not more so, since it constitutes the real support of the structure, and the greater its depth, the higher the building.

In the upbuild of the voice there is a series of tones which are of the lowest pitch, and of limited sounding power; they nevertheless form the cornerstone in the formation of the voice. These tones which carry the low part of the compass of the voice to its physiological limit can be formed only by the minimum of breath and the minimum of tension of the vocal cords; thus they create a natural and easy mechanism of voice production by establishing a preliminary adjustment of the vocal cords which will rule throughout the entire range of the voice.

When these preliminary low and feeble sounds are gradually succeeded by a series of tones higher in pitch and louder, the voice production has the advantage of finding itself placed on a correct basis which will remain throughout unless the vocal organs become affected by artificial influences capable of changing their original adjustments.

With this mechanism the voice acquires a larger range, because according to the laws of acoustics the larger the size of the instrument, the less air is used in producing sounds, and the lower is the pitch of the resulting tone. By using little breath, therefore; and by keeping the vocal organs in complete relaxation, thereby enlarging the vocal instrument to the utmost, a range of lower extension is created. This is the lowest physiological limit of the natural range of the voice.

Singers who carelessly cultivate the habit of forcing their tone production from the beginning of their training acquire a mechanism which shortens the range of their voices, besides depriving them of the invaluable support of the lower part of their natural range, which is the solid foundation in the upbuild of the singing voice. Their voices, consequently, have no more resistance than houses built on sand.

The natural range of the voice, therefore, constitutes a number of progressive sounds, extending from the lowest to the highest pitch of the voice, when produced by a correct vocal mechanism. To guarantee these sounds a correct formation, it is imperative that the tension of the vocal cords during their various adjustments, and the amount of breath required for producing them, work in harmonious accord. By complying with these rules the resulting mechanism of voice production is controlled by the minimum tension of the vocal cords and the minimum breath released by the lungs.

It is also obvious that the vocal cords, in increasing their tension and shortening their length for producing higher pitches, come under a physiological control which guarantees that their adjustments are made with almost unnoticeably increased power, thus avoiding forced and sharp singing. Therefore, to produce correct voice mechanism, both the moving and producing power must be governed in their coöperative work by the fundamental law—the minimum of energy for the maximum of efficiency, since voices based on this law are free from effort, and nearest to perfection.

Another important factor in voice production is the necessity for the tones to reach the mouth unhampered, where they are to be transformed into full voice. The laryngeal sounds must travel freely through the larynx and pharynx with their original number of vibrations, so that they may get the advantage of a resonance proportional to the entire volume of their vibrations.

This is of prime importance, for if the laryngeal vibrations are hindered from freely taking on the resonating power, they produce a voice of poor quality, thin in volume and feeble.

The causes for this interference in the delivery of the voice, though most serious, have never been given due importance. The contraction of the larynx and pharynx, the stiffening of the tongue

and palate, and foremost the bending of the epiglottis over the opening of the larynx are the aforementioned causes which hinder the vibrations from
coming forward.

As a result of these interferences, the section of
the vocal apparatus extending from the trachea to
the lips is reduced in size, becoming narrower and
causing the most appalling defect in voice production.

According to the rules of acoustics as applied
to resonating tubes, the pitch of the tone becomes
higher as the size of the tube is reduced in width.
Therefore in the case of the vocal apparatus—the
most perfect sounding tube because of its power
of elasticity—its exaggerated contraction brings
about an alteration in the pitch of the tone. The
elastic property of the vocal apparatus which enables it to establish a perfect control of its dimensions should be utilized in a normal way during the
adjustments of the vocal organs in producing the
different tones of the range, avoiding any exaggeration in the rhythm of the vocal mechanism.
As a matter of fact the adaptation of the vocal
apparatus should be so gradual as to be almost involuntary on the part of the singer. The great
prima donna, Emmy Destinn, questioned by the
author years ago about her sensations while singing,
said: "When I sing I feel as if I have no throat."
This statement proclaims the most wonderful and
instructive truth about voice production.

An easy mechanism of voice production enables
the larynx to produce free and full tones without

strain, and allows it to rely on the constant coöperative assistance of the moving power which can supply any amount of breath necessary for producing
and carrying the sounding waves to the resonating
power.

Lowering the epiglottis over the opening of the
larynx, however, and stiffening and contracting the
tongue and palate, which bring about a partial
obstruction of the opening of the pharynx, constitute such marked obstacles to the freedom of the
tone that they must not be overlooked.

Singing teachers and experts on voice have
neglected to illustrate the correct functioning of
these organs in voice production, due perhaps to
the fact that through a misconception of the vocal
mechanism the breathing apparatus and vocal cords
have almost monopolized their entire attention,
much to the detriment of voice culture.

Researches and publications dealing with the
breath and the function of the vocal cords are
countless; yet in spite of all the elaborated discus-
sions and suggestions for methods of breathing,
diaphragm development, and tone production, bad
singing prevails at present more than in any other
epoch. It now becomes imperative to establish the
exact status of the rôles played by these organs in
the mechanism of the voice, so that they may be
placed at their proper valuation in voice culture.

The epiglottis is a flexible cartilage which, by
shutting the opening of the larynx, protects the
vocal organs from such foreign bodies as food, or
drink, which would otherwise easily be carried down

into the breathing apparatus during the inspiration. In the process of voice production it has the important function of keeping the laryngeal cavity open for the free passage of the sounds on their way from the vocal cords to the mouth.

Picturing the epiglottis as a door for the larynx, its sole function is to remain open during the respiratory and vocal process, and to close during the passage of food and drink, or, in other words, during the act of swallowing.

For our purpose, however, it is important to illustrate its function only in relation to the voice mechanism, in which its position, whether erect or inclined toward the opening of the larynx, establishes a difference of result in the voice produced which is worthy of the most careful consideration.

When the epiglottis stands erect (Fig. 9), or bends toward the larynx (Fig. 10), being attached to t h e b a s e of the tongue, it is closely connected with all its movements, and their relationship, in voice production, of decisive consequence. In swallowing, the epiglottis must bend toward the larynx, thus closing its

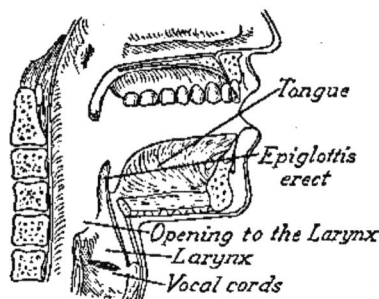

FIG. 9.—THE EPIGLOTTIS ERECT

opening and preventing food from getting into the breathing apparatus. The tongue helps this movement by contracting its base and pushing the epiglottis backward and downward. When the act of swallowing is over, both organs resume their former position, the epiglottis standing erect, and the tongue lying relaxed on the floor of the mouth (Fig. 10). This position is the natural one for singing; but things are merely reversed by a defective voice production, which substitutes the mechanism of swallowing for that of singing. This erroneous function cannot be the physiological one, as it is evident that in order to have the full number of vibrations carried to the resonating power a large opening of the throat—possibly the largest—must be formed.

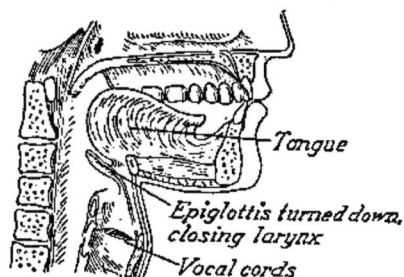

FIG. 10.—THE EPIGLOTTIS TURNED DOWN

The interference of these two organs is so commonplace that very few singers escape its influence. In most cases the tongue—the very worst enemy of singers—is actually the responsible factor, because by its contraction it exerts such pressure on the epiglottis that the latter is forced down toward the opening of the larynx. Therefore the narrow space existing between the epiglottis and the pharynx becomes still narrower, thus choking and preventing a large number of vibrations from reaching the resonance chambers. This condition starts the original disorder, which brings about the disequilibrium in the mechanism of voice production.

It seems that an instinctive influence—the result of a nervous reaction or misinterpretation of the mechanism of voice production—prompts singers to barricade the back of their mouth when they begin to sing. They start by contracting their laryngeal organs as if in self-defense against an imaginary enemy—the sound—holding also all parts of their body in a tense and rigid position.

The vocal cords, thus reduced in size by the contraction of the larynx, produce forced sounds which are greatly hampered from reaching the chambers of resonance by the lowering of the epiglottis, and by the contraction of the base of the tongue. Thus, most of the sounding waves remain confined to the larynx alone for their resonance. This implies first that the voice is centered out of its natural focus, the mouth, and is therefore misplaced; also that the vibrations are prevented from getting their natural expansion and from reaching the resonance chambers.

After this disorder takes place, it consequently follows that the pressure of the breathing apparatus, which acts under the same nervous influence and erroneous conception as the mechanism of singing, becomes more powerful. Then the vocal struggle commences.

The larynx, reacting to the violent blast of breath, increases its tension, and produces a voice decidedly sharp and thin. The singer, worried about his deficient vocal results, tries to improve them by increasing the breath. It is like adding more fuel to a fire that is already smothered by too much of it. The more breath the singer adds, the tighter the vocal organs become; the more his voice fails to show results, the more convinced he becomes that he is not giving enough breath. Thus a vicious circle is established.

Then all the resources of elaborated methods of breathing and diaphragm support, and the most strenuous laryngeal adjustments are put into action. The lungs become a blowing machine, and the vocal cords, under the violent blast of air, hardly succeed in controlling the rhythm of their vibrations. The congestion of the singer's face bears evidence of the painful efforts and the struggle he is making. The muscles, blood-vessels, and nerves of his neck stand out in ugly prominence, making the performance more painful. As a climax to these ineffectual efforts, the big and anticipated effect bursts out and is usually embodied in a strangled whistle very similar to that of a rusty locomotive. Our Latin ancestors would say: "Parturiunt montes ridiculus mus nascitur!" ("Mountains burst and a ridiculous mouse is born.")

This is the average spectacle which audiences are called upon to witness in the singing of to-day, when, because of these false methods, voices fail by the hundreds, and singers whose natural gifts would entitle them to a long and glorious career are compelled to abandon singing after a few years of painful struggle and devote themselves, in most cases, to the profession of teaching.

Yet to say that correct singing, capable of carrying out beautifully all human sentiments in spontaneous form, is a very simple function, is to state a physiological truth. It is certain that if nature

were left alone to govern the mechanism of voice
by her physiological rules, without the profane
interference of incongruous theories and methods,
a natural form of singing based on scientific truths
would now exist, and would be the real guarantee
for correct voice culture. Students must remember
that every error at the beginning of their training
becomes a permanent habit in the future singing.

When the tone, by its complete freedom, suc-
ceeds in getting into the domain of the resonating
power, another important factor completes its full
formation.   All of its characteristics—volume,
quality, loudness, etc.—which are connected with
the property of resonance, lend to the resulting
voice their enriching power. We will treat this
great advantage later, in a special chapter, devoted
to resonance and its most important contributions
to voice production.

An original view also about the rule played by
the breath in voice culture, which is a conception
almost entirely in opposition to most theories about
the mission of the breath in singing, will be treated
at length in the following chapter.

It must be stated, however, that the freedom of
the tone represents the fundamental pillar on which
the correct mechanism of voice production is built.

CHAPTER XI

THIRD PRINCIPLE

BREATH is an indispensable factor in voice production, but *it is not* the essential power which develops the voice as it is taught to-day. On the contrary, the function of singing develops the breathing apparatus and its power, just as any physiological function develops the organ from which it takes origin. Therefore, *singing* develops *breathing*, not *breathing*, singing.

The suggestion that any one who wants to learn piano playing, dancing, skating, fencing or any other sport should first undergo special training for the development of his fingers, arms or legs would undoubtedly seem preposterous. The same false principle, nevertheless, when related to the art of singing, does not give rise to any objection. On the contrary, the artificial training of the breathing apparatus for the purpose of learning to sing is such a commonplace practice at the present time in the teaching field that all kinds of physical exercises for developing the muscles of respiration and the chest are urged in most books on voice. It would rather seem that the singing students were being prepared for an athletic career.

The author, much interested in the teaching methods prevailing nowadays has frequently questioned beginners regarding the kind of vocal exercises they were taught in their preliminary work, and has often been informed that their training was confined principally to breathing maneuvers for the development of the diaphragm and breathing apparatus. In one instance the student, a young man of twenty-five years, told that his teacher was making him sing scales for an hour a day, saying: "*he, he, he,*" and that peculiar exercise had been indulged in for nine months under the supervision of this well-known teacher in New York for the sole purpose of strengthening the diaphragm, so that the pupil could put his breathing apparatus in form for further voice training.

This is by no means the strangest method advocated by singing teachers. From another pupil we have learned of the "*umbrella method,*" which consists in opening the umbrella for the expansion of the chest and closing it during the inspiration. Enrico Caruso, while commenting on these methods, told the writer of a teacher who had his pupils lie flat on the floor and breathe while he was piling a specific number of bricks on their chest. By increasing their number gradually, thus putting a severe test on the resistance of the pupil's chest, the teacher would measure the progress made each time.

It seems ludicrous that grotesque performances of this kind are still going on in the studios of many teachers in our days of progress and evolution when science has revolutionized our life with the most astonishing discoveries.

Independently, however, of these considerations, the fact that breathing is a physiological function brings this subject into the field of science, which alone can establish well-defined rules of physiology in reference to the act of singing. The rules of physiology and no others must be in charge of the function of breathing during the process of voice production.

We remember having read this invaluable statement in a book on singing: "He sings best who attains the best results with the least expenditure of energy." It could be advantageously completed by adding: "He sings the longest who forces his voice the least."

Breath in voice production is unquestionably a most important factor; but its importance must be properly appraised and considered more in the light of *breath distribution* for attaining an artistic style of singing, than in that of force. The principal error of the many voice experts and teachers is that they totally disregard, when it comes to voice production, the fundamental law of physiology that governs all human functions: "the minimum of energy for the maximum of efficiency."

The amount of energy developed by a human organ in order to produce a certain action constitutes what is called a *physiological function*. This amount should be the minimum the organ can produce, and the result should be the maximum of efficiency as related to the energy employed. This balanced relationship between power and efficiency constitutes the *normal function* of an active organ, and establishes the correct mechanism of every organic function.

Applying this principle to the physiological mechanism of breathing in voice production, it is evident that the minimum of breath which is capable of putting in vibration the vocal cords and generating sufficient sound vibrations for producing the different tones of the vocal range, constitutes the *normal amount required* for the correct function of singing.

This establishes the fundamental relationship between the moving power—the breath, and the producing power—the larynx.

From this principle we derive the very important deduction that only the *normal* breath has the physiological property of producing correct tones; in other words, scientifically, only the normal breath can give the exact number of vibrations necessary to produce a tone in its exact pitch, and in its normal volume, loudness, and quality. A surplus of breath, by increasing the number of vibrations of the tone, alters the pitch and the aforementioned dimensions—volume, quality, and loudness.

Another fact that has been discarded in general is the evident danger of exposing the voice to physical deterioration by using the breath under high pressure, for, were it recognized, its employment would be radically modified.

No real advantage, under any circumstances, can result from use of the voice under high pressure, just as no advantage can accrue to a fencer from using his arm under a terrific strain.

In every wind instrument, oboe, clarinet, flute, etc., the expert player employs an amount of breath rather small compared with that of the inexperienced player; and the tone of the instrument is much larger and more melodious in the former case than in the latter. The instrument itself, if played always under high pressure, deteriorates easily and lasts but a few years; after some time of strenuous use no sound can be gotten out of it unless a tremendous amount of breath is spent. The same happens with pianos after years of hard pounding.

In the vocal apparatus these conditions are more manifest. In fact, by blowing forcibly into an ordinary wooden or metal instrument its walls, being rigid, do not react; while in the vocal instrument the muscles and cartilages of the throat, and above all the vocal cords can be very much affected by the violent stroke of the blast of air. The throat reacting becomes very tense, and the vocal cords under the exaggerated pressure cannot produce their vibrations normally, since their movements are not coördinate, equal and balanced, for lack of proper control.

When the vibrations of the vocal cords are not equal, synchronous and balanced, they cannot, according to the laws of acoustics, produce perfect tones, because this condition establishes the decisive difference between tone and noise. The voice, therefore, produced under high pressure, approaches in quality rather a noisy sound than a distinct tone and loses all the characteristics attached to its natural beauty, besides being out of the scientifically correct pitch. The result is that the efforts and large expenditure of energy used by singers serve the sole purpose of deforming and wasting what nature provided in a correct form—the precious gift of a beautiful voice.

From this fundamental fault many others of psychological nature originate, all of which combine to make of the most spontaneous and easy act of singing a very difficult and dangerous function. The fatal consequences are the deformity and the deterioration of the vocal organs, which are destined to wear out more easily than any wind instrument.

The fact that many singers force their voices with the idea of getting better results invites this question: Do they realize that they are forcing? Do they foresee the disastrous consequences which they are inviting by doing so?

Usually *not*. As a matter of fact any remark made to them to the effect that they are abusing their vocal organs is always emphatically denied; they assure you that they *are not using* any force; that their singing is the easiest and most spontaneous action. Meanwhile they are giving full evidence that they have not voice enough left for making this explanation convincing—a peculiar and unfortunate psychology! An intoxicated person, while trying to stand on his feet, always persists in saying, "Do you think I am drunk?"

Thus we find this class of singers always ready

to make an emphatic show of the expansion of their chests, and to parade around asking people *to feel with their own hands* the resistance of their diaphragm; and while their strenuous singing is a real effort they do not hesitate to say that it comes to them most naturally.

These singers see only the spring of their careers and vanish before the summer.

What is responsible for this absence of self-judgment?

A little thought brings about this conclusion. The mechanism of voice production which these singers, by discarding natural laws, employ under high pressure of breath, establishes from the very outset of their voice education a false background of rules and theories on which their psychological conception of singing is formed. Adding to this the faulty training which gradually deteriorates their vocal organs by exercises of an injurious nature, it is inevitable that the wrong foundation becomes the natural standard of voice production for these students who are to be the future singers.

On the other hand, the fact that they have never been accustomed to a normal production of tones makes them unaware of the difference between their voice production and the correct one.

Therefore, they can never see their own defects, just as the ragtime player, while he bangs heavily on the piano, cannot see the difference between his playing and the delicate touch of a refined interpreter of Chopin.

The real responsibility for the false conception of the important part breath control plays in the production of the voice rests entirely with the incompetent teachers of to-day, whose methods are based on erroneous principles.

The absurd and unnatural use of the breathing apparatus, and especially the *magic* power centered on the diaphragm, constitute the true cause of so much bad singing nowadays. The few celebrities of the singing stage we possess offer us the best evidence against these erroneous methods.

If it were true that the power of breath and the strength of the diaphragm play such an important part in the mechanism of voice production, what would happen to those who are not endowed with such physical resources of large proportions? It would seem that those of small stature and of delicate structure would be deprived of great vocal production.

Bonci, for instance, is one of our greatest and most correct singers, whose breath has never failed to assist him in his artistic delivery; yet everybody knows that Bonci is not built like an athlete.

It is a strange coincidence that many coloratura sopranos and lyric tenors who sing mostly in the upper tones of the range and who, according to the theories in vogue, should require a huge amount of breath and terrific strength of the diaphragm for the support of their sustained tones, happen to be rather undeveloped physically and oftentimes have not even the power of breath resistance given to the average person. We can cite the case of a world-famous coloratura soprano, very frail and delicate, who startled the musical world with an instantaneous success, and whose breath never failed her in the most difficult executions of her coloratura variations. On the other hand, we could name a large number of strongly developed singers, with large chest expansion, whose voices are painfully poor and insufficient. Taking into consideration their physical appearance, their developed lungs, muscles of respiration and all other organs related to the vocal apparatus, these athletic specimens could offer no excuse for the insufficiency of their voice if it were true that voice production depends so much on the strength of breath.

It is evidently untrue that with the aid of physical equipment capable of producing a large amount of breath, or with a particularly well-developed diaphragm a singer is endowed with the indispensable assets for good voice production. This false theory, which unfortunately is almost universal to-day, can hardly be defied without offending the traditional feelings of the faithful believer in the diaphragm's almighty power! Furthermore, this erroneous principle has so influenced the musical world that even those outside the singing field, such as some music critics and dilettanti, have set the power of breath and the strength of the diaphragm as a standard in appraising the value of an operatic or concert singer. "Short of breath," "diaphragm support," "strength of breath" are the usual epithets employed in the discussion of artists and their singing merits.

Even the great Caruso has not escaped the application of this false standard of judgment; he whose phenomenally sustained tones were not the result of a strenuous breath power but of a marvelously balanced distribution of it which enabled him to indulge in his most striking effects.

The greatest singers of the past knew very little indeed about the diaphragm and the mechanism of voice production in general; still their names remain revered in the memories of music lovers. I believe that most of our best contemporary singers have only the vaguest notion of the physical mechanism of the voice, but they are not to be reproached as long as their singing conforms with natural laws.

The following incident has been related to us by a prominent American soprano. The famous Adelina Patti was visiting the studio of a world-renowned singer and teacher in Paris to hear some of his pupils. After one of the students, who had been cautioned by the professor as to the use of his diaphragm, had finished singing, Patti turned to the teacher and very candidly inquired, "Well, what is that diaphragm? I never heard of it during my career." This is one of the most striking remarks made by an indisputable authority in confirmation of our theory.

In the fields of Italy the author has heard the peasants—while they work at picking olives or grapes from the ground—sing in a chorus their popular folk songs, as is their custom. Among them he could detect some soprano voices reaching such high pitch that it was almost inconceivable to imagine that human voices could attain such altitudes. Yet these natural singers were kneeling on the ground in a cramped position, and, judging from the beauty and the ease of their voices, wonderful and blessed seemed the absence of theories and methods about the use of the diaphragm in singing. Their voice production was physiologically as perfect as it was unconscious, and I am sure that the diaphragm-apostles of the teaching fraternity of to-day would feel doubtful about their theories had they the opportunity to hear them.

Here, in New York, a little boy eleven years of age, born of poor parents, was discovered by an American physician, who, while passing through one of the streets of the lower East side, was attracted by a beautiful voice coming from one of the crowded tenements. The physician made inquiries about the possessor of the beautiful voice and was greatly astounded when he was presented to a tiny, underdeveloped lad. The same evening the child was presented to the writer, who, looking at the tiny singer, concluded that the matter of his voice had been exaggerated by the enthusiastic discoverer. He asked the child what he could sing. "Pagliacci, Martha, Rigoletto," was the unexpected answer. Who taught you to sing?" "Caruso . . . on the phonograph," he answered. And the child, taking the floor like an experienced tenor, sang

one after another of the most difficult arias from the
above-mentioned operas, with a big resonant voice,
in which the natural sentiment and pathos were not
secondary to the dramatic force and expression
suggested to the child by the powerful singing of
his teacher—Caruso.

During the wonderful and touching performance
of this little singer one could not refrain from a
sense of pity for those mighty disciples of a *trained
diaphragm,* who, while trying in vain to produce
perhaps one-half the amount of voice of that minia-
ture tenor, look almost ready to explode like rubber
balloons.

What then, is this concern about the breath?
Why the need of such long training for the artificial development of the diaphragm?

Breathing is a natural function, independent
even of our own will. We cannot prevent breathing. Let nature, then, take care of this function;
she will provide for it when necessity presents itself. Let nature suggest or rather carry out her
own mechanism of breathing, and let us not attempt
to interfere with it and deform it.

We breathe all the time, whether awake, asleep
or unconscious. Our very life is dependent on this
providential function and we have no reason to
think of it. *Why then should we devote so much
thought to it when singing?*

Of course we must discriminate between *force*
of breath and *skill* of distribution. If more attention and effort were given to the latter a proper
conception of the mechanism of singing would be

obtained. The singer who after a few tones is compelled to take another breath does not know how
to distribute his breath, even though he may be an
expert in breathing and in the art of using his
highly trained diaphragm.

On the other hand, the singer who knows how to
distribute his breath never runs short of it, and the
normal respiration furnishes him enough power
with no cause to worry about the strength of his
diaphragm or his intercostal muscles. Nature helps
him in the most exceptional instances, such as exist
in certain operatic arias where a surplus of air is
necessary to produce dramatic effects, coloratura
variations and long cadenzas. Caruso's singing in
the "Pagliacci" aria was the typical demonstration
of this statement.

Our conception about the all important factor—
the moving power—in the mechanism of voice production discards all theories and suggestions related
to the different types of breathing, such as the
clavicular costal or abdominal respiration because
we believe that the student of singing should not
be conscious while performing this natural function of life. The physiological respiration, which
we employ from our birth, is the natural one, and
it must also rule our breathing when we are singing.

The beginner who applies to a teacher for assistance in voice culture, and is put under the shame-
ful training of artificial means for developing his
breathing apparatus like a circus athlete, and whose
mind is fed on the absurdity that the secret of good

singing lies in the strength of his breath and the power of his diaphragm, is misled at the very outset of his career, and is given a false foundation. He invariably loses the spontaneous conception of singing, which usually is given by nature itself as a compliment of her gift of a beautiful voice. It should, therefore, be left to nature to take care of her own product—the voice—and if the student is endowed with intelligence and a marked musical sense he does not need any artificial help other than a guiding hand to watch his development and to keep him always under the control of natural laws. The guiding hand should be the teacher and nothing artificial should be substituted for nature itself.

The strength of the breath and its volume in singing must be the result of a correct mechanism of voice production; by the *prolonged but normal* employment of breath the muscles of respiration become naturally stronger and gradually increase their power of resistance. This system alone, after years of voice training and a singing career, will acquire that perfect control which is one of the fundamental pillars of correct singing. Practically the same thing will happen as in the case of dancing, fencing, or any other physical sport.

The physiological laws of respiration, therefore, must be the sole rules to follow, and all false notions about the artificial development of the respiratory organs must be discarded as dangerous by those who aspire to a successful vocal career.

CHAPTER XII

Resonance is the *most important factor* in voice production. It furnishes to the voice volume and quality, and emphasizes its loudness. To *rely* on *resonance rather* than on *force* is essential for producing a big and pleasing voice.

To understand the phenomenon of resonance, it is indispensable to become acquainted with the few laws of acoustics, which are most closely related to it. The readers, however, who desire to get a more complete knowledge of this interesting property of sound, can refer to any treaties on acoustics where this subject is widely discussed.

In order to explain what resonance is, we prefer a practical rather than a scientific illustration, since it is more advantageous for our purpose.

A common experience—talking into a megaphone—shows how the voice can become greatly magnified in its characteristics—loudness, volume, and quality. This is merely the result of a resounding property furnished by the horn of the megaphone.

If we hold a violin string by its extremities, in tension, against a brick wall, or an empty space, and strike it, an almost imperceptible sound develops, given by the vibrations of the string. If

100

we put the string on an empty case—wooden, metallic, or of some other material—the sound becomes much louder and more resonant. The reason is that the amount of air contained in the empty case vibrates also under the stroke of the vibrations transmitted by the string, thus magnifying the vibrations in number and amplitude. The sound, so decidedly enlarged, is the result of the string only, in so far as the embryonic element, the vibrations, is concerned; the case is responsible for its development and enlargement.

The auxiliary function of the megaphone and of the case, with their characteristic power of magnifying the original vibrations of the sound constitutes what we call *resonance*.

In the human voice the sounds, as produced by the vocal cords, are weak and colorless, but when magnified by the resonance furnished by the laryngopharyngeal and oral tube, plus the resonance chambers and body cavities, they become larger in volume, stronger in loudness, and of softer quality.

The laryngopharyngeal cavity and the mouth—a natural horn—as compared with the megaphone —an artificial horn—act as a resonating apparatus which magnifies the rudimental vibrations of the vocal cords into full voice, just as the megaphone makes the sounds produced into it more voluminous. In both cases the decided improvement in their original vibrations is due to the intervention of the magnifying power of resonance.

Scientifically, a tone produced without resonance is a simple sound; with resonance it becomes a compound or complex sound. The original sounds produced by the vocal cords are simple, made up of vibrations of limited sounding power. They become complex when enriched with the resonating power of the body cavities which gives them timbre, volume, and loudness. We say *body cavities,* because we venture to assert that the human body, in all its cavities, acts as a big resonator for the voice.

Although a chest and masque resonance, originating from the chest, the antrum and frontal sinuses, are generally admitted, up to the present time no mention has been made of the body resonance. Nevertheless if, according to the laws of acoustics, the vibrations travel in every direction, provided they are not intercepted by any obstacle, there is no reason why the sounding waves should stop at the aforementioned cavities of the chest and masque instead of spreading all over the body, getting the resonance of all its other cavities—the head, bones, abdomen, and joints combined.

What usually interferes with the transmission of the sounding waves from the larynx to the body, confining the radius of their expansion to the nearest cavities is caused in most cases by a throaty production which checks the expansion of the voice.

As a result of this false mechanism of voice production even the amount of resonance given by the nearest cavities is sometimes obliterated also, as the exaggerated contraction of the throat prevents the sounds from reaching the resonance chambers. If this is true of the nearest cavities, it is logical to suppose that interferences of similar nature are likely to prevent the vibrations from reaching the more remote sections of the body, thus hindering the cavities of these sections from making the valuable contribution of their resonance.

The rigidity of the muscles of the body, for instance, which is usually the coefficient of a forced mechanism of voice production, and an instinctive act with many defective singers, represents a marked physical obstacle to the traveling of the sound vibrations.

A simple demonstration of this can be obtained by following closely the phenomenon of resonance in musical instruments. A piano, for instance, improves its tone merely by being placed on a wooden platform, in which state its vibrations are not confined to its strings alone, nor to its case. They travel in every direction and are transmitted even to the floor and walls of the room, from which they get other vibrations and resonance, if the material of which they are composed has resonating power. Piling many articles of heavy material on the piano and playing it on a tiled floor, or even on a floor covered with thick carpets, are sufficient causes for markedly diminishing the power of its resonance.

All opera houses and theaters are constructed according to the rules of the physical property of expansion of the vibrations and their resonating power. Architects take particular pains to obtain the best acoustics by scientific methods, which guarantee the free expansion of the sound waves, so they can reach any empty space within the walls of the building, which are constructed of such material and in such a shape as to produce new vibrations, thus increasing their power of resonance.

As for the human instrument, a well-built body, with all its strong bones and large cavities, undoubtedly furnishes one more factor of resonance to the resonating power, which should not be neglected.

There are singers who stand rigidly and heavily while singing, and their stiffness creates such an obstacle even to the circulation of the blood, as to be easily discernible in their spasmodic expressions, and in the congestion of blood in their faces and necks. These singers undoubtedly deprive the voice of most of its resonance, because the rigidity of their muscles and tissues prevents the spreading of the sound vibrations from the source of their production to the entire body, just as it prevents the blood from running freely all through the circulating system.

Several years ago, a prominent London doctor startled the entire musical world by saying that Caruso possessed musical bones.

A certain newspaper in New York solicited interviews with some laryngologists to inquire into the possibility of possessing musical bones. The writer was one of those consulted, and he found it most difficult to convince the interviewer that, although there are in truth no musical bones, there is a possibility of human beings possessing organs made of tissues of exceptional resonating property, which is dependent, perhaps, on the quality and constructive essence of the cells from which they are made.

Indeed, Caruso had no musical bones; but the writer can affirm, from personal knowledge, that they had a power of resonance which was startling. In fact, by tapping on his mastoid with a finger, or, as he did himself, with his ear lobe, a sound was produced which could be heard at a considerable distance. This represented merely the exceptional power of resonance of his bones, which were composed of very fine, compact resounding matter. This is not at all surprising when we consider that in some musical instruments the kind of wood from which they are made has a striking influence on the resonance of the tones produced, the quality and volume of which, according to manufacturers, is even related to the number of years of seasoning of the wood. The hypothesis is naturally suggested that the compactness of the cells and fibers of certain trees has the characteristic property of lending to their wood a more remarkable power or resonance.

Why can not this same possibility exist in the human body? The resounding property of the masque, head, chest, etc., which are hollow cavities surrounded by hard compact matter, may be dependent upon the nature of the cells, which constitute the constructive substance of the entire frame of the body.

This subject is worthy of a certain scientific consideration, and should arouse at least sufficient interest for finding out whether the privilege that certain races possess, of having a greater number of beautiful voices, is not attached to some physiological property dependent upon their method of living, alimentation, climate, etc., which creates a certain difference in the anatomical structure of the tissues of their bodies.

The soil, sunshine, air, light etc., which are responsible for making the fibers of certain trees hardier, drier, and of more compact matter, better fit for the bodies of musical instruments than others of soft and spongy nature, raised in marshy, damp fields, constitute the characteristic conditions which influence the different growth of those trees. Cannot the same natural conditions have some influence upon the physiological development of the human tissues of the inhabitants of certain regions? By a logical deduction, this should be so. Of course we are not talking of beautiful voices in reference to their phonetic and artistic qualities; as for singing, we must not discard the fact that the more marked aptitude of certain races for expressing their feelings through singing is due to psychological influence, such as musical education, environment, temperament, and, principally, hereditary disposition. We think, though, that even these traditional racial qualities have at the bottom a physiological ground, which was generated primarily by the above-mentioned natural conditions, and evolved gradually into a psychological form from generation to generation, for centuries. The temperament of the Latin races, for instance, especially the Italians, has always been associated with a certain influence of the mild climate, the bright sunshine, the clear skies, the volcanos, etc., all such elements which seem to be responsible for some of their characteristics and natural dispositions, and have undoubtedly influenced the psychology of that race.

Therefore, the author's hypothesis has some scientific and material foundation. The human body contributes resonance from all its cavities, and there may exist a difference in the quantity and the quality of resonance in different persons, which is dependent upon the constitutional structure and the development of their tissues, and perhaps upon the origin of their races.

The voice has three characteristics which are closely allied with its power of resonance: loudness, timbre or quality, and volume. From the combination of all of them a strong, beautiful and resonant voice results.

A recent view, already quoted in this book, gives to the resonance the power of producing vocal vibrations, besides the function of magnifying them, a function which is generally attributed to the vocal cords alone. Thus, according to this view, the *resonance* plays a more *important* rôle, combining both the power of *magnifying* and that of *producing* sound elements.

The vibrations, by their power of expansion, spread from the vocal cords into the larynx, where certain resonance is given to the fundamental sounds by the ventricles of Morgagni. They then expand through the pharynx, all over the mouth, the resonance chambers and the entire body. In the resonance chambers more vibrations are produced by those already traveling from the larynx, all of them becoming reinforced in their dimensions and characteristics by the resonating power. This coördinated strength, resulting from the intensity and amplitude of the vibrations produced by the vocal cords and by the resonance chambers, and their magnified resonance, is responsible for the loudness of the voice, which constitutes the most striking of its characteristics.

The second characteristic of the voice—the more valuable—is the timbre or quality, which to most experts signify the same thing. It is the author's view that the quality or timbre of the voice possessing the distinct property of pleasing the ear constitutes the most prominent characteristic in voice production. It is worth finding out, therefore, what physical factor gives quality to the voice.

If we strike a tone on the piano, and let the sound fade gradually, toward the end of its vibrations, we hear a series of lighter tones which are perfectly harmonious with the original, though much higher in pitch. The tone we hear so distinctly at the beginning, which fades gradually, after a while, is the *fundamental* tone, which we are playing. The other sounds, which are concomitant tones to the fundamental one, are the so-called *overtones*. The fundamental tone is the lowest in pitch but much stronger than the others; the overtones are higher and much softer, and are to the tones what the shadows in a painting are to the drawing. A well-trained ear can detect the overtones in voices correctly produced, while in voices produced by a forced mechanism only the fundamental tone can be heard, or certain high overtones which do not entirely harmonize with the fundamental one.

Voices produced with only fundamental tones are poor in quality and *dry,* lacking the richness in overtones; those in which incorrect overtones prevail are disagreeable and decidedly forced.

The quality of the voice can be enriched only through the abundance of its correct overtones. Because of their importance, therefore it is of interest to know their position with regard to the fundamental tones.

The most important overtones are located on the octave, the twelfth, the fifteenth, and the seventeenth notes of the fundamental tone. Striking a note on the piano, C below the staff, for example, the first overtone is C of the next octave; the second overtone is G above the staff, which is five notes higher than the first and twelve notes higher than the fundamental tone. The third overtone is high C above the staff, fifteen notes higher than the fundamental one; and the fourth overtone is E, which is seventeen notes higher than the fundamental tone; and so on.

There are higher overtones, in addition to these, but they are difficult to detect, except with the aid of Helmholtz resonators, and are of no help in singing, therefore useless to discuss.

According to Helmholtz, the overtones which are perceptible to the ear are those which determine the quality of the voice. Their presence or absence, whether partial or entire together with their intensity, decides the particular characteristic of the organ, whether more or less metallic, and gives to the voice its distinctive quality.

The overtones are so intimately connected with the fundamental tone that to change their number or intensity means to change its quality. In fact, as we said before, a sound without overtones is soft and sweet, but feeble, small, poor; with the lower overtones—those classified above—the sound becomes rich, harmonious and full, still retaining its softness, if all overtones are produced with the same proportional intensity.

In voice production, when the overtones over the fifth become more prominent than the fundamental tone, the voice becomes sharp and disagreeable. Those overtones which should be ignored are, on the contrary, much developed by the current methods of singing, based essentially on the force of the breathing apparatus, which emphasizes, by an exaggerated number of vibrations, only the highest overtones.

The fullness of the voice is due to the prevailing intensity of the fundamental tone in relation to its overtones. On the contrary, the dominating intensity of the overtones over the fundamental tone causes an emptiness in the voice, which is the result of thin, small vibrations. The presence, therefore, of the overtones, and their relative position toward the fundamental tone, is of capital importance in relation to the most beautiful of its characteristics —the quality.

The contribution of resonance to the volume of
the voice is of much greater importance than that
furnished by the moving power—the breath, or by
the size of the vocal cords—the producing power.

In musical instruments the volume of the tone is
dependent principally on the size of the case of resonance, which is related to the amount of air it
contains, and to a certain extent also to the quality
of material of which it is made. The larger and
finer the wooden body of a violin, the larger the
volume of its tone. The tone of a violoncello is, in
fact, bigger than that of a violin, due more to its
larger case of resonance than because its strings are
thicker, although this has some bearing also on the
volume of the tone. All the foregoing proves that
the size of the vocal cords in relation to the volume
of voice is of much less importance than the amount
of resonance which can be given by the resonating
power.

As for the moving power—the breath—it cannot
be compared with the power of resonance. Increasing the power of a violin bow for the purpose of producing bigger tones cannot compare with the improvement gained by giving to the violin a Stradivarius body, so rich in resonance. The strings of
the Stradivarius, when put on another violin, fail
to give the same tone, even in the skillful hands of
the greatest virtuoso. All of this proves how important is the rôle played by the resonance and its
physical properties in all musical instruments.

In the human instrument the volume of the voice
is related to the size of all the cavities of the body,

the quality of its tissues perhaps having some relation too.

The chest and resonance chambers, with the antrum and frontal sinuses, being the nearest cavities to the source of the voice, have a more decided influence on its resonance so that those in whom these organs are well developed have the best conditions for producing the largest amount of resonance.

The shape of the palate also has a very marked influence on the resonating power of the voice. A well-arched palate enlarges the oral space for the sounds, and has the same acoustic property as the vault of a bridge where even small voices are intensely magnified by, perhaps, new vibrations created by the vault itself. For the same reason the tongue has some effect on the resonance.

Titta Ruffo, the world-famous baritone, has told the writer of a singer whose voice was mediocre, but who could shape his tongue in a decidedly concave position like a cradle, thus creating a larger oral cavity for the resonance of his voice, with remarkable results. Evidently the instinctive conception of that singer was correct, for, by shaping his tongue in this position, enlarging the space, he created more resonance for his voice.

This should serve as warning to the many singers who hold their tongues in a stiff and contracted position, thus abolishing most of the mouth's precious space. The illustration in Fig. 11 gives practical evidence of how the tongue should be shaped to create the largest space and resonance in the oral cavity.

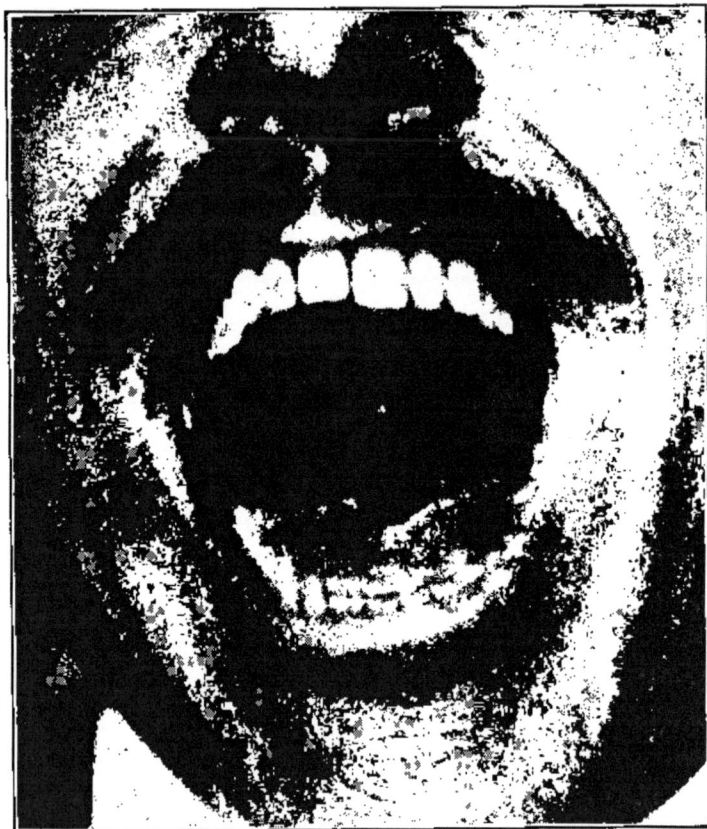

Fig. 11.—The tongue in complete relaxation on the floor of the mouth, and in a concave position to create a larger space in the oral cavity

All the author's efforts in the foregoing pages tend to show that Resonance is the most important factor in voice production.

To rely on *resonance,* and not on *force,* must be the aim of every singer; and to remember that the largest amount of resonance can be obtained only by the complete relaxation of the vocal organs, must be the fundamental rule of any method of voice culture. The methods in vogue, which base their foundation on breath, that is, on force, are as erroneous as dangerous.

CHAPTER XIII

Speaking and *singing* are *similar functions,* produced by the same physiological mechanism; therefore they are the same vocal phenomenon.

The speaking voice acts as the substantial factor of the singing voice and constitutes its real support. Singing, in its very essence, is merely speaking in musical rhythm; hence no correct singing can exist without a correctly produced speaking voice.

Voice is speech made up of words formed of vowels and consonants. In its complete form voice comprises two like phases, similar and closely connected, though slightly different in the degree of their intensity and effect; one is related to speaking, the other to singing.

Scientifically, however, there is no difference between the speaking and the singing voice as physiological phenomena, both being produced by the same vocal organs with an identical mechanism; nor is there any difference in their phonetic elements, except that singing is emphasized by musical colors.

The speaking voice prepares the words for the singing voice, which adds to them the beauty of rhythmic melody. Vocal principles and rules referring to one must logically apply to the other.

The idea of claiming an intimate physiological relationship between the speaking and the singing voice is not new, as many writers on voice have given more or less attention to this subject. But its vital importance in relation to voice production has been entirely overlooked thus far, or underestimated to such an extent as greatly to have hampered the progress of voice culture.

To us, however, it represents a factor of the most essential and inestimable value, since it constitutes the platform on which our method of producing and placing the voice is based. It is, therefore, our earnest desire to call the attention of voice experts to this subject, so as to create a deeper interest in the close connection existing between these two intimately related forms of the same physical element which constitutes the human voice.

Fundamentally, speaking and singing are produced by the same physiological mechanism. They are both formed by the coöperation of the moving, producing, and resonating power, though the vocal organs act with more efficiency when the singing voice is concerned, and whether in speaking or in singing it is to the medium of phonetic expressions --words—that we have recourse to express our ideas or sentiments.

In the fusion of these two elements, the speaking voice constitutes the material part, the backbone or the basis of the singing; consequently it cannot be disassociated in the mechanism of singing, otherwise, by losing its support, the latter would be deprived of its substantial element. In fact, the physical phenomenon—voice—is preceded first by the material act of speaking, and followed by the complementary and decorative one of singing.

The sounds as produced by the vocal cords, if prevented from being transformed into words cannot express anything but physical tones. It is obvious then, that in singing the *psychological* mission of expressing our feelings is entrusted to words and not to sounds, and these words can be furnished only by the speaking voice through the myriad combinations of vowels and consonants. Thus, since no other element but the speaking voice is able to produce them, it is but logical that the basis of the singing voice is the speaking voice.

To give a practical, though rough demonstration of the relationship of the speaking voice with the singing voice, we must think of the former as something material, which serves as the underlying support for the latter and constitutes its substantial intrinsic power during the act of singing. It may be said that it represents the raw and solid elements of the phenomenon—voice—to which singing adds the psychological adornment and finish, through its musical rhythms and colors, just as in a beautifully finished palace the steel skeleton and brick walls constitute the solid, material support of the building, whereas the ornamental finish, in the form of artistic decorations, lends style to the palatial edifice.

Therefore, since the rôle played by the speaking voice in the mechanism of singing is of such essential importance, its correct production is the most indispensable factor and asset for creating a beautiful singing voice. It is the corner stone on which the foundation of correct singing is built.

In cases in which the relationship between these two forms of the same element is disturbed, the singing voice is always the one which suffers. In fact, a deformed and disagreeable speaking voice can never develop into a correct and pleasing singing voice, because, being its intrinsic factor it cannot avoid lending to singing its defects as well as its beautiful characteristics, when they exist.

Cases in which the singing voice proves different and more agreeable than the speaking voice are those in which the latter is so falsely produced as to be entirely deprived of all its natural qualities. Likewise, cases in which the speaking voice is correctly produced, and the singing voice is defective, are those in which the latter is not molded on the former, thereby losing all the advantages it would derive from it.

It occasionally happens that the speaking and singing voices are produced by the same individual independently of each other, as in the case of singers who unconsciously talk with one voice and sing with an entirely different one. In such cases either the singing voice is artificial, being composed of only the original sounds of the vocal cords before they are transformed into voice (a falsetto voice), or the speaking voice is produced by a very defective mechanism, which becomes improved during the act of singing.

At any rate, if the mechanism of voice production in singing loses its fundamental relationship with the speaking voice, it is almost impossible to prevent the tones from being produced in the throat, which constitutes the most appalling defect known as throaty production.

Artists who sing with this method never succeed in making the audience understand their words. In fact, remarks like, "His voice is so throaty;" "He (or she) sings so badly, in his throat;" "I don't understand a word he sings," are very frequently heard in the audience, and it is unnecessary to emphasize that even the general impression of the layman is that a voice produced in the throat is entirely misplaced and ugly.

Theories or practice, therefore, which bring about a throaty production are fallacious, and are responsible for the worst defects in voice production.

The erroneous principle that *sounds* are the central element in singing has been presented in many books and enforced by many methods of singing, proving a dangerous influence in voice culture. These methods, by discarding natural production, are compelled to resort to elaborated technicalities in order to compensate for the deficiencies of the voice resulting from its misplacement and faulty production. Therefore, all the gymnastics of the voice, and the many kinds of muscular exercises inflicted upon pupils, with the idea that they constitute the proper and physiological ground for voice culture and create an efficient mechanism of singing are ridiculous contrivances, fit rather for an acrobatic education than for students of the art of singing.

In a book dedicated by a singing teacher to her twenty-nine hundred pupils, we find this statement: "It is a positive fact that the voice is in the throat. . . . When a maestro says to a pupil who emits a bad tone, 'Don't sing from the throat,' he makes a wrong statement, as we must necessarily sing from the throat, nature having placed the larynx in the throat. If he were to say, 'Don't press or squeeze the throat,' he would speak more correctly."

Evidently this singing teacher bases her remark on the belief that the larynx is the real center of the voice, which is not true, and makes no discrimination whatever between sound and actual voice.

While it is true that we produce *sounds* with the throat, we must *not* necessarily sing from the throat, if we are to obey the laws of natural mechanism of voice production which place the voice in the *mouth*. The mere precaution not to squeeze the throat does not prevent the defect of producing the voice in the throat. That can be accomplished only by giving to the throat the sole attribute of forming the sounds and leaving to the mouth the function of transforming them into voice. The author is insistent on this subject, because a throaty production destroys entirely the innate connection of the speaking with the singing voice, thereby creating a condition contrary to physiological laws.

The falsity of all the vocal theories identified

with physical training is obvious. The throat has only the physical power of producing sounds, and even these must be the result of an easy mechanism so as not to cause any disagreeable sensation or ill effect to the throat of the singer. These sounds, being only the germ of the voice, are naturally poor tones, which cannot be compared with the resonant phenomenon of voice as completed in its full form in the mouth and enriched by the coöperation of the resonance chambers.

In a résumé we wish to state emphatically that the speaking voice, as the physical basis of the singing voice, is also its psychological medium for expressing emotions and consequently constitutes its natural element for building up both a correct and an artistic method of singing. It is merely a law of nature that we cannot disregard the support of the speaking voice in the production of the singing voice. Speaking beautifully and resonantly, in fact, is equivalent to singing, without musical rhythm, and with less brilliancy and color. Sarah Bernhardt, Eleonora Duse, and many other celebrated dramatic artists have given full evidence of this statement.

The speaking voice, when correctly and beautifully produced, lending to singing its substantial element in the form of words made up of vowels and consonants, makes us think of the well-shaped stones of a mosaic, which, being equal, smooth and artistically arranged, make of the mosaic a perfect work of art. The singing composed of beautifully spoken words bends toward artistic perfection.

Hence, going to the very root of voice production, only by forming correct and euphonic vowels and consonants can a correct and artistic method of singing be established.

By making of the speaking voice the leader and guide of the singing voice, the words become the essential elements on which singing is built. Therefore a singing voice molded on the speaking voice gains the advantage of taking over all its attributes, characteristics, and qualities.

In the singing of that master of song, Enrico Caruso, one of the most striking features was his rendition of the so-called "recitative" of the operas. His "recitative"—the nearest thing to melodious talking—was the clearest, most colorful and brilliant display of what a valuable coöperator the speaking voice is in singing. He gave more delight to the world, and raised more emotions with his musical speaking than many singers with their big or pure tones, which, no matter how pure or big, are far from reproducing the real human voice. Human voice is made of vocal color expressing human pathos, a characteristic which is absent when producing tones, as in the case of a musical instrument. Human pathos was the magic power of Caruso's voice, that voice which penetrated to the innermost depths of the souls of all those who have had the good fortune to hear him.

CHAPTER XIV

The *pitch* and the *dimensions* of the singing *voice*—the *volume*, the *quality*, and *loudness*—are determined by the *speaking voice*. Speaking *high* or *low, resonant, loud* or *soft,* in any gradation of sentiment and shade of color, lays the ground for singing in *high* or *low* pitch, *loud, resonant* or *soft,* in any musical color and expression.

In a previous chapter it has been demonstrated that fundamentally there is no difference between the speaking and the singing voice. Likewise no difference can exist in their dimensions.

The speaking and the singing voice being a similar phonetic act of the same function, their pitches and dimensions must stand in the same fundamental relationship. The speaking voice, which constitutes the purely physical element of the voice, furnishes to the pitch the raw material to which the singing voice—the artistic element—lends the musical character and color.

By talking high or low, or in any intermediate *altitude* of the speaking voice, we produce its various pitches. If our talking is rhythmical and the vocal vibrations are equivalent in number to those required for producing the different notes of the musical scale, the pitches we determine are exactly the same as those of the singing voice. Talking, then, ceases to be "speech" and becomes "singing."

It is generally agreed at present among scientists that the pitch of the voice is determined by the number of vibrations given by the vocal cords. These vibrations, reinforced by the resonating power, determine also, in addition to the pitch, the loudness, volume, and quality of the voice, all the physical properties called the dimensions of sound.

The author's views on this subject are partly different and this difference is of basic importance, as it affects the theory we have demonstrated in our First Principle, that *voice* and sound are not exactly the same thing and consequently their *pitches* are not the same either.

As in singing we aim to express our feeling through *words,* it should be the concern of voice experts to find out what the pitch of the *words,* that is, voice, is rather than that of the sounds.

The sounds become voice after a phonetic transformation in the mouth; their pitch, therefore, as determined by the number of vibrations of the vocal cords only, represents only the pitch of the *laryngeal* sounds, in which is lacking the phonetic support of the words. When these tones materialize into words and are transformed into the speaking voice, their pitches, produced by the *ensemble* of physical functions that form the voice, become the pitches of the singing voice.

It is obvious, then, that the same difference that distinguishes the sound from the voice also exists between the pitch of the sound and the pitch of the voice. This consideration is of the greatest importance in voice production, as it devolves upon the speaking voice the task of determining the pitch.

Dr. Scripture has already aroused doubts about the existing theories of the pitch by demonstrating, through experiments based on the transmission of the vibrations of the vocal cords, that the pitch is also determined by the vibrations of the resonance chambers which are set in vibration by the sound waves coming from the larynx.

Dr. Scripture's new point of view has aroused interest among voice experts, and we notice that it has been indorsed by no less an authority than Dr. Mills, who, in his book on voice, says: "To Prof. Scripture belongs the credit of demonstrating that the resonance chambers determine pitch also," and later on: "Such views have become more widely known, and it is hoped that, as they are very radical, they may be established by other methods."

Dr. Scripture's theory, however, differs from ours in the same respect as those of other experts, inasmuch as he too treats of the pitch and the dimensions of the *sound* instead of the *voice*.

According to our conception, which relies on the speaking voice for the determination of the pitch, any of its altitudes constitutes the intrinsic basis for the corresponding pitch of the singing voice. The vocal cords, however, by furnishing the vibrations for the embryonic sound, determine its pitch in the *embryonic form;* the more the vibrations the higher the sound. But the *real* pitch of the voice

is established by the various altitudes reached by
the words, when the vibrations are transformed in
the mouth into voice. Speaking *high* or *low,* or
in any other degree of the range, constitutes the
true pitch; it has the true substance of voice-quality
and not the shrill characteristics of a whistling
sound.

Those who never gave much attention to the innate similarity of the speaking and singing voice
cannot think of the possibility of an analogous
pitch quality, volume and loudness for both, having
the impression that, in speaking, voices cannot be
raised to as high a pitch as in singing, and that
loud, voluminous voices cannot be produced in
speaking. This belief is erroneous and is contra-
dicted both scientifically and practically.

The great variety of inflections resorted to by
great orators and dramatic artists in order to bring
out striking effects or to emphasize the meaning
of certain words is dependent upon a large range
of pitches and a richness of color and shades.[1] Talking in falsetto, imitating the voices of singers,
women or children is nothing else than producing
the various pitches which naturally exist in our
voices but are not used.

In reality the use of different pitches in talking
is very much neglected in general, except among
the Latin races, who inherit with their languages
and their vivacious temperaments, the natural dis-

[1]Ancient orators used to give so much coloring of speech to the inflection of their voices that they gave the impression of singing their orations.

position for warmth and color in their speech; their voices, therefore, possess naturally the flexibility of the different pitches.

We cannot help remarking that this natural cold, colorless and almost monotonous way of speaking is highly detrimental when singers and dramatic artists are concerned. The advantages of a well-modulated speaking voice are of inestimable value in the dramatic as well as in the lyric art, as no other natural gift has the psychological power and influence of a beautiful speaking or singing voice to reach the depth of a human heart. Artists like Tommaso Salvini, Eleonora Duse and Sarah Bernhardt have realized it; in this country we may mention Julia Marlowe, Julia Arthur, and a few others. To attain superior success these artists first availed themselves of the most important element of the art—their voices. It is to the exceptional coloring of her voice—her most striking asset—that Sarah Bernhardt owes the largest share of her fame.

The various nuances of the speaking voice, with all the gradations of its pitches, give the true expression of life to all the emotions of human psychology—love, sorrow or joy, without the aid of music, but almost in the same keys as in the singing voice. The fact that insufficient consideration is given to the great importance of voice modulation by the dramatic profession of this country is to be highly regretted, as undoubtedly the lack of life, brilliancy and expression in the speaking voices of most of the actors on the American stage can be ascribed as one of the main reasons for the monot-

ony and the rudimentary heaviness that character-
ize the American dramatic art of to-day. Educated
audiences tire of them and with good reason; nobody cares to listen for hours at a stretch to the
monotonous and uniform voices of actors in which
the spice of the coloring and intonations given by
varying pitches is almost totally lacking, just as
very few would care to look at a sky constantly
blue or to travel through prairies monotonously flat
without a hill or a tree.

These same artists could achieve better results
by educating their voices in the use of different
pitches than by struggling for sensational effects
obtained by growling or roaring spasmodically in
their throats.

It is of great advantage, therefore, to take into
consideration the importance of cultivating the
pitches of the speaking voice, as they are of the
utmost assistance in the dramatic art and also of
inestimable value in the formation of the pitches
in the singing voice.

The dimensions of the voice—volume, quality
and loudness—like the pitch, originate with the
speaking voice and are transferred to the singing
voice. We think it preferable and more precise to
designate these dimensions as the *characteristics of
the voice,* because they represent the essential attributes which differentiate voice from sound and
even one voice from another.

The characteristics of the voice, which are less
prominent in speaking merely because they are not
emphasized enough, become distinctly marked in

singing, when the moving, producing, and resonating power are compelled to coöperate with higher efficiency under the strong psychological influence of the music.

We can, therefore, consider the pitch and the dimensions of the *singing voice* as determined by the number, length, amplitude, and intensity of the vibrations of the vocal cords augmented in number and improved in quality by the resonating power; but *ruled entirely* by the psychological influence of the words.

This statement will meet with objections; but it is the author's conviction that if we were to rely on the pitch and the dimensions of the sound as produced by the vibrations of the vocal cords alone, the quality, volume, and loudness of the sounds would be proportioned to their very limited sounding power, and would consequently be detrimental to the voice. In other words, the voice would be thin, poor, and insufficient, as the producing power of the vocal cords is actually of so little value in the emission of rich and ample sounds that it would almost be impossible to conceive of the existence of resonant and strong voices were the efficiency and the strength of the vocal cords to be considered as the only factor.

The author calls the attention of the reader to one more point, which tends to show that the determination of the pitch cannot be confined only to the number of vibrations given by the vocal cords. The idea is based on the law of acoustics relative to the resonating tubes.

The altitude (pitch) of a sound produced by resonating tubes is proportional to their size; the smaller the tube, the higher the pitch.

Applying this law to the human resonating tube we see that as long as the sounds produced by the vocal cords are kept within the space of the larynx, they are ruled in their pitch only by the number of vibrations of the vocal cords, and by the resonance they get within that organ. But as soon as they reach the pharynx on their way to the mouth, the resonance chambers and the lower cavities, in their expansion toward the chest, by getting into a tube of larger size they undergo a physical change in pitch, which is similar to the change in tone produced by substituting a resonating tube of larger size for one smaller. The pitch becomes somewhat lower. The human resonating tube, being composed of elastic tissues—the lungs, trachea, larynx, pharynx—and movable tissues—the mouth with the tongue, palate, lips—is apt to change easily in size. By this change the original laryngeal sounds can be altered in their pitches, becoming higher or lower, according to the change in size to which the vocal organs adjust themselves. This shows that the privilege of determining the pitch of the voice cannot belong entirely to the number of vibrations produced by the vocal cords; there are other physical properties of the sound, related to the other parts of the vocal apparatus, which are concerned also. In fact, to give a practical example, if, in producing a tone in the human tube, we contract the throat and close the mouth, and then gradually relax the former and open the latter, we hear a certain difference in the pitch of the tone, without having altered the number of its vibrations, however.

The same experiment can be made by singing or whistling a tone into the cavity formed by the palms of both hands, while they are held close together only on their outer edges, thus creating the largest space possible. By contracting them gradually and reducing the space inside, or *vice versa,* while producing the tone, a change of pitch is perceived which evidently is not related to any increase in the number of vibrations, but only to the increase or decrease in the amount of space created by the hands.

These experiments should induce singers not to diminish the size and dimensions of their vocal organs, by contracting them, if they wish to keep their voices in their natural form. It is true that in singing higher tones the vocal organs adjust themselves to a smaller size, but this adjustment is almost imperceptible, and is purely instinctive and involuntary, and must not, therefore, be artificially exaggerated by a conscious influence, which most of the time is the result of an erroneous conception of voice production.

Condensing in one illustration the relationship of the pitch of the sound with the pitch of the voice, we conceive of the first as the germ, from which the second takes origin and develops. In its fundamental essence, the pitch of the voice is the pitch of the sound, but it is not exactly the same thing, as in its formation are included, besides the vibrations produced by the vocal cords, perhaps some new vibrations created by the resonance chambers. If no new vibrations are created, though it is certain that the original ones of the sound are largely emphasized in size, length and intensity, bringing about a decided, if not a radical, change in the dimensions of the pitch, which becomes comparatively larger, louder and more powerful, and all the characteristics of the voice, such as volume, quality, and, to a certain extent, loudness, are more prominently displayed with it.

The following sketch gives a rough idea of this relationship:

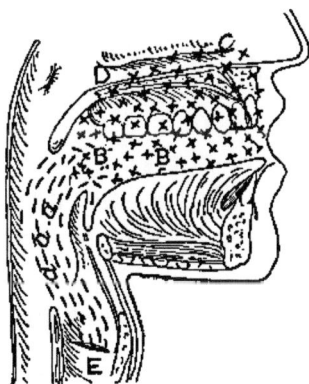

aaa. The sound and the *sound waves* going through the pharynx on their way to mouth. Pitch of sound is shown here in its original form as determined by the number of vibrations of the vocal cords. Its dimensions exist in their embryonic form. This is the first phase of voice production

C. Voice. Voice contains within itself the sound.
D. The pitch of the voice which includes the pitch of the sound, plus the vibrations created by the resonance chambers. The volume and quality of voice are very prominent in this second phase of voice production
E. The vocal cords

B. *Sound,* in its original pitch after reaching mouth to be transformed into voice

FIG. 12.—THE RELATION OF THE PITCH OF THE SOUND WITH THE PITCH OF THE VOICE

The real conception of the pitch, then, can be summed up as follows:

Sound is the result of the vibrations of the vocal cords, and is confined to the laryngeal cavity. Its pitch is related to the number of these vibrations, and is merely a *sound* pitch, lacking the dimensions of the voice, in quality and in volume.

Voice is the result of the sound produced by the vocal cords, reinforced through its phonetic change into full voice, by the vibrations of the resonating power. Its pitch is related to the vibrations of the vocal cords, plus the vibrations of the chambers of resonance. The embryonic sound produced in a determined pitch, if it is transmitted freely to the mouth, is transformed into real voice, and retains its pitch, enriched by the resonating power of the mouth and of the resonance chambers. The resonating power establishes for the voice its characteristics: volume, quality, loudness, etc., and determines also its real pitch in every tone of its range. All of this mechanism is ruled by the speaking voice and transferred to the singing voice, the speaking lending to the singing its pitches, its characteristics or dimensions in their normal degree, and the singing emphasizing them.

In voice culture the determination of the pitch by the speaking voice, especially in raising the voice to high altitudes, brings such surprising advantages as to render worthy of consideration the adoption of rules for making the speaking voice the guiding element for producing high pitches in singing.

No doubt the difficult task of reaching the high tones has always been to singers *la bête noire* of their careers. Yet, we contend, this difficult problem can be solved satisfactorily by using the speaking voice as the medium for reaching high pitches.

A rough demonstration can be given by this practical experiment. After reciting a phrase distinctly in a low pitch, sing it immediately in the same pitch. A musically educated ear can very easily ascertain the similarity of pitch. Then, raising the pitch of the speaking voice to some point at about the middle of the range of the voice, recite and then sing the phrase in the same pitch. Finally, raising the pitch gradually, continue up to the highest pitch possible for the speaking voice, and place the singing voice at the same height.

It is surprising what results can be obtained by this process. Even the highest pitches of the singing voice will present no difficulties when their production is performed along the track of the speaking voice. Singers who cannot conceive of the possibility of reaching certain high tones will be astonished at the results of this experiment, which is made possible only because the singing voice is carried to its high altitudes through the speaking voice, by placing the pitch of the former on the pitch of the latter.

In the first act of "Aïda," the closing phrase of the famous aria, "Celeste Aïda," "*Un trono vicino al sol*"— a difficult task for any tenor because of its high pitch—if spoken first at its approximate altitude, and then sung at the same height, proves easy when compared with the usual rule of attempting that pitch by means of the singing voice alone.

Thus through this method great elasticity can be given to the singing voice in making its pitch, while, if singers attempt to raise their voices merely by forcing the sounds produced by the vocal cords, discarding the auxiliary help of the speaking voice, they will always find great difficulty in reaching their much coveted B flats or high C's.

The misconception about the pitch of the voice is responsible for this difficulty, and by giving to the speaking voice the task of determining the pitch it will positively disappear. The speaking voice is the real mold of the singing voice, in all its characteristics and dimensions; therefore, it must also be the factor for its different pitches.

CHAPTER XV

THERE are no *registers* in the singing voice, when it is correctly produced. According to natural laws the voice is made up of only *one* register, which constitutes its entire range.

According to almost general understanding the singing voice, at certain points of the natural range, breaks into series of tones and gives origin to the so-called registers of the voice.

Some writers contend that there are four or five registers; but the great majority of them claim only three, and this classification is universally adopted by singing teachers. A few authorities, however—among them Sir Morell Mackenzie, the well-known English laryngologist—admit two physical changes in voice production, while only a very small number of voice experts agree on the existence of but *one* register. It must be said that in none of these instances are these divisions founded upon a concrete or definite scientific truth.

The teachers who uphold the division of the voice in three registers call them the chest, the middle, and the head registers.

The author contends that no such division is suggested by nature, nor is it needed in voice culture. The breaks of the voice are the result of abrupt and artificial changes in the laryngeal adjustments when the vocal organs are adapting themselves to produce higher tones; the normal function of these organs is then disturbed and a defective vocal production is thus brought about. In fact not only is this classification not essential or necessary, but it places the mechanism of voice production at a certain disadvantage.

If we make an incidental analysis of it we are at first striken by the incongruous designation of the registers as chest, head, and middle. It is obvious that in speaking of the chest and head registers, reference is made to the resonance obtained by emphasizing the voice in the chest and head cavities. What about the middle register then? To what cavity does it allude?

The supposition that it would be a *pharyngeal* register would imply that the resonance is confined in the pharynx, which would give a *throaty* voice production, the most appalling defect in singing.

Another current misunderstanding exists in reference to the head register, which sometimes is confused with the so-called *mezza voce*. There is a substantial difference between them, which it is important to establish *a priori,* so that the criticism leveled at the head register may not be extended to the *mezza voce*.

When a singer is called upon to give his entire volume and intensity of voice in any part of its range for dramatic effect, he carries to the higher tones the same proportional volume and intensity of voice with the same quality, and this constitutes a dramatic style of singing in full voice; it can only be obtained by avoiding the break of the voice into registers.

But when the meaning of the words and the style of the music require lyric and delicate effects, only part of the voice—the *mezza voce*—is employed, being better adapted to express artistically and truthfully the meaning of words set to lyric music.

Caruso—a dramatic as well as a lyric tenor—in singing dramatic rôles used his full voice, in lyric parts the same voice but in lighter form, which in certain soft passages was very similar to a *mezza voce*. His correct mechanism of voice production made it possible for him to resort to the most perfect lyric style of singing without changing the intrinsic nature of his voice.

Singing in the *mezza voce* is then physiologically correct since it is performed without changing the mechanism of the *full voice*, with only this difference, that less intensity is used, while the volume and the quality of the voice remain the same.

There exists, then, a substantial difference between the *head register* and the *mezza voce*, which should be better understood.

The empiricism and the confusion that rule the singing field are put in relief by these commonplace and elementary errors; yet these are only a few of the many examples that go to explain the stagnant and chaotic condition of the art of singing as it is to-day.

Sir Morell Mackenzie, who wrote the most interesting book on the hygiene of the voice, admits, as previously stated, only two registers, and calls them the *long* or *chest,* and the *short* or *head* registers. This classification is by far more rational than all the others, and is based on the resonance of the chest for the long, and of the head for the short, register.

With all due respect to so great an authority, we venture to analyze this division as compared with the theory of *no* registers, except for the natural range; and we advance the following hypothesis:

Dr. Mackenzie defines the registers as a series of tones of like quality produced by a particular adjustment of the vocal cords.

According to this definition, the voice being divided into two registers, the chest register of a soprano singer, for instance would extend from low C to medium E, and would be represented by a series of tones of like quality produced by a *particular adjustment* of the vocal cords.

Following this there would be another series of tones produced by another adjustment of the vocal cords, with tones different in dimension than in the first series, and this would represent the head register.

Now, what can justify this change of the vocal cords to a second adjustment? Must it be attributed to a natural law dictating this alteration in the mechanism of voice production, or to an incorrect use of the vocal apparatus, particularly of the producing and moving power, which make this change in the mechanism of voice production unavoidable?

No concrete reason has been given by Dr. Mac-kenzie for his classification. In fact further on he admits that, strictly speaking, there should be a different register for every note, which practically coincides with the theory generally accepted, that slight changes must take place in the vocal organs during their progressive adjustments for the ascending tones of the scale. But these gradual adjustments are not the same as contended by register advocates, according to whom the registers are originated by marked changes in the shape of the vocal organs in certain sections of the range where the voice breaks. There is no objection to having as many progressive registers as there are notes in the range, because practically it is tanta-mount to having one big register made up of as many small registers as there are notes in the com-pass of the voice, like one long chain formed by a great number of small links.

Therefore, Dr. Mackenzie's classification, hav-ing no definite scientific basis, remains purely a personal view, which, however, stands out promi-nently among the many others as the most logical.

Dr. F. E. Miller, in his book *The Voice,* after illustrating the theory on registers, states that the breaks of the voice can be accounted for on scien-tific grounds:

Suppose [he says] there were a man able to produce the entire male vocal compass, from deepest bass to highest tenor. While for every note throughout the entire compass there would be subtle changes in the adjustment of the vocal tract the following also would be true: that beginning with the lowest note and throughout the first octave of his voice, the changes in the adjustments of the vocal tract would not alter the general character of the adjustment for that octave; that on entering the second octave, there would be a tendency toward change in the general adjustment of the vocal tract; while for the production of the remaining notes above, an almost startling change in the adjustment of the vocal tract would take place.

As much as we respect the opinion expressed in the above statement, we fail to perceive the scientific ground which justifies the necessity of the breaks of the voice into registers.

That slight changes of the vocal tract must occur in passing from one tone to the next, when the vocal organs undergo different adjustments for producing progressive pitches, has been demonstrated by scientific experiments and is admitted by all scientists. But that there is a tendency toward a change in the general adjustment of the vocal tract on entering the second octave, and that, for the production of the remaining notes above that, a startling change must take place in the adjustment of the vocal organs, has not thus far been reinforced by any scientific evidence.

And if it were true that the change in registers must occur at a certain particular altitude of the scale, it has not been demonstrated, up to this time, that this altitude is the correct place. There are singers, in fact, whose voices break in any difficult passage, and others—very few—whose voices never break through the entire range. We cannot think otherwise, then, that the division of the voice into registers, far from being a scientific axiom, is nothing else than an arbitrary and conventional hypothesis of voice experts, teachers and singers, who do not even agree among themselves as to where the breaks of the voice should occur.

Now and then [Dr. Miller adds] in a generation there may appear upon the scene a singer, usually a tenor, who for his high notes is not obliged to adopt the somewhat artificial adjustment required by the highest register, but can sing all his tones in the easier adjustments of the lowest or middle register. But he is a phenomenon, the exception that proves the rule, . . .

This privilege which Dr. Miller claims for one singer *in a generation* is not so rare, we venture to say, and is far from being exceptional. As a matter of fact it is *the rule* with singers who produce their voice correctly, and furthermore, it should be the universal practice in voice training, as it is in absolute conformity with the normal physiological mechanism of the vocal organs.

Nature, as a rule, creates perfection through simplicity; the simpler the mechanism, the smoother and the more perfect its function; we can, therefore, hardly credit Nature with the complications that occur in the break of the voice into registers, and which we maintain are only the result of improper singing; neither can we think that Nature would bestow upon a few chosen singers physiological privileges which are denied to the generality. We are rather inclined to think that as in the case of blood circulation—the simplest and most wonderful function of the human system—the natural mechanism of voice production is one and the same for all of us.

Those singers whom Dr. Miller considers as "phenomena" are nothing more than good singers, conspicuous only through their scarcity and the deficiency of the others. Their great merit lies in the knowledge—whether conscious or unconscious —of how to make use of their vocal organs according to the laws of Nature.

Duprez, for instance [quotes Dr. Miller in his book] was a phenomenal tenor; he could sing the whole tenor range in the chest register. He could emit the *ut de poitrine,* which means that he could sing tenor high C in the chest register.

But there are others: Caruso could sing basso, baritone, dramatic and lyric tenor, without any breaks in his voice, and we believe he was not an exception in this. Of course, there was a slight change in Caruso's voice when he used to sing as a lyric tenor, which affected only the dimensions of his voice, molded most essentially on the significance of the words and on the style of the music, which, being lyric, required a lighter form of voice than in the dramatic parts.

Lablache, the famous basso, used to sing tenor rôles as well as basso. Emma Calvé, a rare singer as well as exceptional artist, can sing as contralto and coloratura in one and the same voice. Galli-Curci uses only one register for the entire range of her voice, which covers almost three octaves, from G to F, and Titta Ruffo, the brilliant baritone, can invade very gallantly the domain of dramatic tenors with the same voice he uses for his entire range of baritone.

All this is not exceptional; when the vocal organs are properly adjusted for the different tones of the scale, every singer can acquire a voice production without breaks in the vocal range. In the case of many singers the changes of registers take place so frequently that they are condemned as "bad" singers even by people not well versed in the art of singing; the unevenness of their voices is caused by the continuous breaks at different points of the range, and the fact that the popular verdict is against them clearly shows that the public favors those who avoid breaks in their voices. This natural predilection of the uninformed listener is the best proof how essential is the homogeneity of the voice in quality and in volume.

To well-trained ears, the passing of the bow from one string of the violin to another produces somewhat of a peculiar and unpleasant effect which the good violinist tries to avoid, and strives to bring out all the tones alike in quality which procures a more uniform and artistic effect.

This dissonance, almost unavoidable in the violin, is only slight when compared with the disagreeable sensation produced by singers when passing from one register to another. The acoustic effects are obviously against the use of various registers in the human voice. To adapt the vocal organs to abrupt adjustments, which are only the result of artificial efforts to produce voices of different character in the same range, amounts to nothing less than the introduction of a faulty mechanism, which interferes with the natural production of the voice and destroys its beauty.

The singing of the greatest tenor in the annals of song—Caruso—gave the most striking evidence of the advantage of avoiding register breaks, and undoubtedly any singer who produces correctly the entire vocal range with a uniform quality throughout, and without any division into registers, is the nearest specimen to perfection in voice production.

The artificial division of the voice into registers, besides bringing about a complicated mechanism is also impractical and disadvantageous. If we produce, for instance, a tone of low pitch, belonging to the chest register, the resonance of which must be confined to the chest only, we eliminate the valuable support of the resonance of all the other cavities of the body and commit a grave error in voice production. No obstacles of any kind should check the sound waves in expanding from the larynx throughout the entire body, so as to get the benefit of the resonance of all its cavities; no reason, therefore, can justify a "chest" production or any other localization which would prevent the voice from getting its full resonance.

The scientific explanation of the disorder of the vocal organs, responsible for the breaking of the voice into registers, is that the adjustments of these organs for producing the tones are extremely exaggerated by two factors: the first is *psychological,* and is constituted by the spasmodic contraction of the larynx, usually at the mercy of psychological influences, as nervousness, fright, and other emotions, which, instead of a normal relaxation, instill into the muscles and cartilages an exaggerated tension; the second is *physiological,* and is represented by the increase of breath which singers feel they must force into their throats in order to counteract the tension of the vocal apparatus, and in the false belief that the harder they blow the more voice they produce.

From this fatal ignorance the notion of registers has originated probably. Singers, instinctively inclined to magnify their voices by giving more breath than necessary even in the lowest notes of their range, produce tones which are forced and also somewhat higher in pitch.

In progressing up the scale, by increasing the breath, the tones become more forced and sharp, and by persisting in this mechanism of forcing and growing sharper, they eventually reach a point when the normal resistance of the strained vocal organs refuses to lend its assistance any longer, so that the distressed singer is compelled to resort to artificial means in order to compensate for the lessened natural resources of the vocal organs. Then a sudden constriction of the larynx, pharynx, tongue, and soft palate combined reduce the vocal apparatus to a considerably smaller size and render it more apt to produce higher tones, which, however, have no longer the dimensions and the character of the previous ones, as we have demonstrated in a previous chapter.

The result is evident: the more strained and contracted the vocal organs, the smaller the spaces of their cavities become, and consequently the volume of the voice produced is less; the greater the amount of breath employed under exaggerated pressure, the less exact is the resulting pitch of the voice and its original quality.

It is our firm conviction, however, that were the adjustments of the larynx but gradually employed with no constriction of the throat to interfere with the freedom of the tone and with the minimum amount of necessary breath employed, a mechanism would result which could regulate the entire range of the voice without requiring a break into different registers.

A rough illustration of what could be considered a perfect range, without division of registers, would be obtained by comparing the voice with a ladder; the wider part is at its base, and it diminishes in width proportionately as it nears the top. This gradual diminishing, however, does not affect its evenness. The identical evenness should remain in the gradual diminishing of the range of the voice, its lower tones, larger in volume, undergoing a gradual and slight decrease in ascending the scale, without this slight change, however, affecting the quality and evenness of the voice in any altitude of the range.

The illustrations in Figure 13 give material evidence of the breaks of the voice, according to the division of registers, with the last one showing the entire range without any breaks.

The first *illustration in the group of three* represents the average compass of any high voice, that is, a dramatic tenor or a soprano, and shows where the usual breaks into registers occur. These breaks, however, are not the same and not equal in number for every voice. Some singers—the very bad ones —have breaks at almost every other note and sometimes, even in the same note, if long sustained, toward the end their voices slide into a kind of a squeezed sound, indefinite in pitch and disagreeable in effect. A certain great singer used to call these breaks the *tails of the voice.*

This traditional, time-worn divisions of the voice into three registers is explained as follows (referring to letters on the diagram):

   a. The chest register which gets its resonance from the chest. At the altitude of E or F the voice breaks and gives origin to the Middle Register.

   b. The first break of the voice.

   c. The Middle register which, according to some authors, gets its resonance from the pharynx. At the altitude of E it breaks and gives origin to the head register.

   d. The second break of the voice.

   e. The head register, which gets its resonance from the head.

The second illustration in Figure 13 shows the defects of the voice, resulting from its breaks into register, emphasized by colors, and referred to herewith by letters.

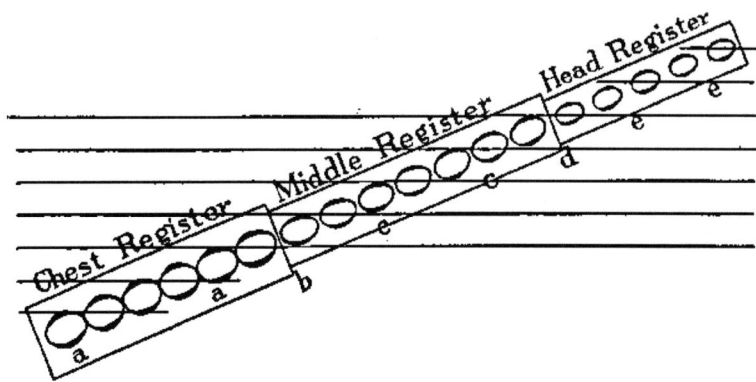

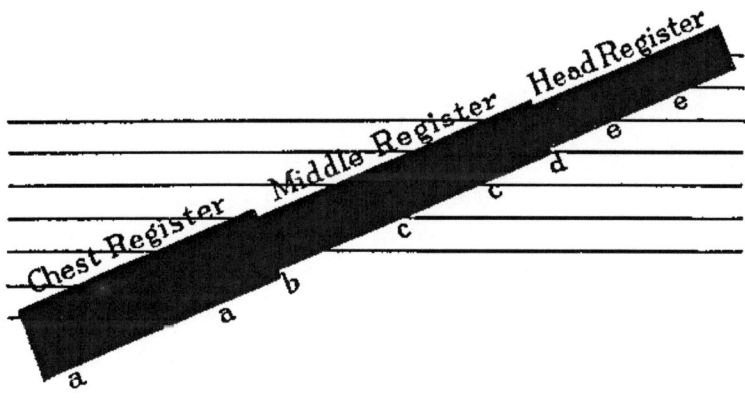

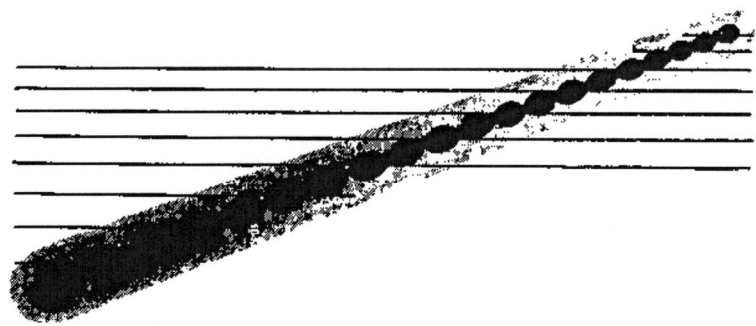

FIG. 13.—VOICE RANGE WITH AND WITHOUT BREAKS INTO REGISTERS

a. Chest register, produced by an exaggerated power and tension.
b. Starting point of the first break. Change in the quality and volume of the voice.
c. Middle register, the voice becomes gradually stiff, thin and sharp.
d. Second break. Second change of the voice, its production becoming more difficult and forced.
e. Head register. The voice becomes very sharp and decidedly changed in its characteristics— volume and quality. Its loses the character of human voice, and sounds like an instrument.

In a faulty voice mechanism, the lower tones being produced by an exaggerated effort for the purpose of getting more volume and resonance, the result is that the vocal apparatus, after a series of a few tones, cannot sustain the tension of its organs, and collapses. The voice breaks and gives origin to another series of tones molded on a new adjustment of the vocal organs, which suddenly reshape themselves into a smaller size, and produce smaller tones. Thus, from the chest register suddenly comes out the middle register, smaller in size (Fig. 13).

The middle register begins to show the deformities of the characteristics of the voice, which grow with the ascendency of its altitude. The volume begins to diminish, and the quality becomes stiff and sharp. From the collapse of the vocal organs at a certain point of the middle register, the head register takes origin.

In the head register the deformity of the voice is more appalling. It becomes empty and colorless with certain singers, or very sharp, though thinner in volume, and more like a sound than a human voice—a kind of a big, strong falsetto. In many instances singers cannot pronounce their words in this register, and therefore confine their efforts to singing tones only.

The third illustration in Figure 13 shows the full range of the voice as performed by a natural, correct mechanism. The lower tones, being produced by a normal amount of breath, can reach the lowest extension of the range, thus enabling the voice to run from E below the staff to high C. These low tones, however, are not strong, but rich, because the complete relaxation of the vocal organs allows their vibrations to expand and get the full resonance from all the body cavities. In singing, however, they are not used by tenors and sopranos.

By gradually ascending the scale there comes a point where the voice becomes naturally strong, without forcing its production, and this represents the natural, brilliant section of the compass, which characterizes the different voices—basso, baritone, tenor, soprano, etc.

The rest of the range of the voice follows the same mechanism, keeping its volume and quality almost entirely. The slight changes which may occur in its characteristics are related to the gradual, slight adjustments of the vocal organs for higher tones, but no breaks whatever into registers can take place.

The voice production with no registers, therefore, is able to render the entire range in the same form and quality, and relieves the vocal organs of any strain, giving also the possibility of training and developing a beautiful voice, with astonishing results.

Were a clear conception of the *natural* range of the voice to exist, nobody would bother about registers. Musical instruments have but one register, and require but one technique for playing at any altitude of their range. Why should it be essential for the human vocal apparatus—the most complete and perfect musical instrument—to undergo an elaborated process of breaks and sudden adjustments for producing the voice?

An original view, of a psychological nature, why we should supplant the theory of registers with one of *psychological intonation* of the voice, is suggested to the author by the fact that the speaking voice through the meaning of the words rules the singing voice and therefore must rule all its modulations in all the altitudes of its range.

The speaking voice has no registers; yet we talk in high and low pitch, and the modulation of our voice, in its different pitches, is dependent upon the psychological influence of the words.

We talk loudly, for instance, when we are excited, angry, etc.; softly and sweetly under the soothing influence of love, joy and tenderness; low on a solemn or sad occasion. All of these psychological phases influence and rule the pitch and color of our voice.

The changes in the character of the singing voice should be, by analogy, related rather to these emotional influences than to the physical mechanism of voice production, and thus render the entire range of the voice equal in form, provided a correct technique is used.

These psychological changes in the altitudes of the tones require no artificial adjustment of the vocal organs. In recitation, for instance, when the artist wishes to express an exquisite sentiment of happiness, tenderness, a dream or a vision, he raises his voice to a very high pitch (some do it very artistically) in order to produce a light and sweet intonation, and diminishing it at times to a mere shadow of a voice. Human psychology could not suggest any other inflection of voice than the high pitch for expressing such sentiments, as for the interpretation of dramatic feelings the medium and low tones are indicated; and the physiological mechanism of voice production fully obeys the psychological suggestion, without, though, changing the intrinsic characteristics of the voice, irrespective of how high or low the pitch may be.

The same must occur in singing; the changes of pitch, correctly produced, must not result in a change of register, but merely represent the psychological color given to the singing by the different sentiments to be expressed. In the unsurpassed love duet of Tristan and Isolde, for instance, it is the beautiful inspiration of the words more than technical execution of the notes that communicates its mellowness to the voices of the interpreters, and the voice production here is less the result of a skillful mechanical function than the corollary of the psychological influence of the words. The "head register" has nothing whatever to do with the light *mezza voce* which is required in this duet and is merely the attenuation of the voice under a psychological influence, just as would be the case if the same words were spoken.

The close relationship of the meaning of words with the altitude of the voice is shown by the fact that sometimes, in phrases of very dramatic portent, high pitches of voice are used, in full power and volume, neglecting entirely the change of the chest register into the more adaptable head register. In the *finale* of the third act of "Aïda," for instance, the tenor holds the words, *Sacerdote, io resto a te,* in full voice, sustaining several high B's, which, according to the division of registers, should be produced by the head register; but in so doing the quality of voice would not be suited to the meaning of the words, and would mar this powerful dramatic situation.

To sum up, there are no physiological needs for the break of the voice into registers; by leaving its intonation under psychological control we can attain any altitude in the vocal compass, without subjecting the vocal organs to artificial efforts in order to break the voice into unnecessary registers.

Let psychology rule the voice within the bounds of one register for its entire range! If singers have drama, tragedy and poetry in their hearts, it will show in their singing, whether tragic, dramatic or lyric. The voice being the product of inspiration and natural resources will certainly be the truest and most beautiful expression of art when free from any artificial influence or deformity like the arbitrary break into registers.

CHAPTER XVI

THE personal opinion of Caruso regarding his vocal method and his point of view on singing in general, besides being of the utmost interest to singers and students of singing, constitutes so great a moral support for this book that the author feels justified in presenting it to the readers before entering into the illustration of the second part of this book.

In 1919, Caruso was requested by a musical paper to give some personal views on singing. The following are the principal points which he explained in the interview and which he represented as the guiding principles of his voice and vocal art:

"The question 'How is it done?' as applied to the art of singing brings up so many different points that it is difficult to know where to begin or how to give a concise idea of the principles controlling the production of the voice and their application to vocal art.

"Every singer or singing master is popularly supposed to have a method by following out which he has come to fame. Yet, if asked to describe the method, many an artist would be at a loss to do so,

155

or would deny that he had any specific method, such a subtle and peculiarly individual matter it is that constitutes the technical part of singing. Most singers—in fact, all of them—do many things in singing habitually, yet so inconspicuously that they could not describe how or why they did them. . . . For instance, a singer will know from trials and experience just the proper position of the tongue and larynx to produce most effectively a certain note on the scale; yet he will have come by this knowledge, not by theory and reasoning, but simply by oft-repeated attempts, and the knowledge he has attained will be valuable to him only, for somebody else would produce the same note equally well, but in quite a different way.

"So one may see that there are actually as many methods as there are singers, and any particular method, even if accurately set forth, might be useless to the person who tried it. This is what I really would reply to any one putting this question to me—that my own particular way of singing, if I have any, is, after all, peculiarly suited to me only, as I have above described.

"However, there are many interesting and valuable things to be said about the voice in a general way. . . .

"It may be well to speak now of a very important point in singing—what is called the 'attack' of the tone. In general this may be described as the relative position of the throat and tongue and the quality of voice as the tone is begun. The most serious fault of many singers is that they attack

the tone either from the chest or the throat. Even
with robust health the finest voice cannot resist this.
This is the reason one sees so many artists who have
made a brilliant début disappear from sight very
soon, or later on wind up a mediocre career.
Singers who use their voices properly should be at
the height of their talents at forty-five, and keep
their voices in full strength and virility up to at
least fifty. At this latter age, or close after, it
would seem well to have earned the right to close
one's career.

"A great artist ought to have the dignity to say
farewell to his public when still in full possession
of his powers, and never let the world apprise him
of his decadence.

"To have the attack true and pure one must con-
sciously try to open the throat not only in front,
but from behind, for the throat is the door through
which the voice must pass, and if it is not sufficiently open it is useless to attempt to get out a full
round tone; also the throat is the outlet and inlet
for the breath, and if it is closed the voice will seek
other channels or return stifled within.

"It must not be imagined that to open the mouth
wide will do the same for the throat. If one is well
versed in the art, one can open the throat perfectly
without a perceptible opening of the mouth, merely
by the power of respiration.

"It is necessary to open the sides of the mouth,
at the same time dropping the chin well, to obtain
a good throat opening. In taking higher notes, of
course, one must open the mouth a little wider, but

for the most part the position of the mouth is that assumed when smiling. It is a good idea to practice opening the throat before a mirror and try to see the palate, as when you show your throat to a doctor. . . .

"The tone once launched, one must think how it may be properly sustained, and this is where the art of breathing is most concerned. The lungs, in the first place, should be thoroughly filled. A tone begun with only half-filled lungs loses half its authority and is very apt to be false in pitch. To take a full breath properly, the chest must be raised at the same moment that the abdomen sinks in. Then with the gradual expulsion of the breath, a contrary movement takes place. . . . It is this ability to take in an adequate supply of breath and to retain it until required that makes, or the contrary, mars, all singing. A singer with a perfect sense of pitch and all the good intentions possible will often sing off the key and bring forth a tone with no vitality to it, distressing to hear, simply for lack of breath control.

"This art of respiration, once acquired, the student has gone a considerable step on the road to Parnassus. . . .

"In the matter of taking high notes one should remember that their purity and ease of production depend very much on the way the preceding notes leading up to them are sung. . . .

"Singers, especially tenors, are very apt to throw the head forward in producing the high notes, and consequently get that throaty, strained voice, which is so disagreeable. To avoid this one should try to keep the supply of breath down as far toward the abdomen as possible, thus maintaining the upper passages to the head quite free for the emission of the voice." [1]

In these few personal remarks on singing, expressed by Caruso, there is more precious advice condensed to help students and singers in their art than could be found in many a book on voice culture filled with abstruse doctrines and complicated rules.

Here the great singer, in a simple and practical form, puts down the fundamental principles of voice production which control the art of singing. By saying that many artists would be at a loss to describe their methods, if they have any, and by emphasizing that most singers do many things through mere force of habit and so spontaneously that they cannot describe how, Caruso has given the clearest possible explanation of his marvelous singing. In his statement that there is no one method of singing, but that there are as many methods as there are singers, and that his own particular way of singing was peculiarly suited to himself, he established the real truth about methods of singing in general. As a matter of fact no two persons can follow precisely the same routine in singing, and not even two pupils can be taught the same method in exactly the same way. This also shows clearly that to try and imitate Caruso's singing was futile

[1] In the *Musical Observer*, November, 1919, taken from the *Monthly Musical Record*.

and perhaps dangerous, as has been proven practically by the attempts made by some tenors, to the great injury of their own voices.

Nevertheless, if Caruso's method of singing could not be readily adopted by any one else, as Caruso himself stated, the practical illustration of the physiological rules of voice production which he followed and on which his singing was naturally molded are undoubtedly of inestimable value to students and singers.

Caruso said that, although he could not explain his method of singing, there were many interesting and valuable things he could say about singing in general. In describing them as he did, he reinforced the scientific truth which he advocated by natural intuition.

As a matter of fact, many of the personal impressions of great singers are often the very fundamental principles of voice production, based on physiological laws, which they follow through mere instinct. The physiological rules which control the production of all voices are like the rules of proportion and perspective governing the drawing of a painting or the modeling of clay. They establish the correct fundamental basis for every individual vocal method. Therefore, while Caruso could not illustrate for others his own method of singing, he almost unconsciously laid down the physiological principles of voice production by deduction from his own experience.

The author had the rare opportunity of assisting Caruso in teaching the only pupil he ever had

—a person with a superb voice, but too advanced in years to be influenced by any training. By closely observing the method by which Caruso taught this man, the author saw the application by the master himself of the correct physiological rules of voice production as propounded in this work.

These rules coincided exactly with the principles presented by the author in this book; thus Caruso's opinions constitute their most valuable confirmation. The laws of natural singing which he, the typical model of natural singing, felt and followed by natural instinct and inspiration, are those that the author claims must be adopted in voice culture. It was not in Caruso's power to formulate his instinctive feelings into practical rules, as he did not have the support of scientific knowledge about voice production, and naturally he was rather at a loss when asked to explain his method of singing.

He was, however, deeply interested in the problems of human voice, and in the many years of friendly association with the author much was discussed on this subject between the great singer, from his personal point of view and experience, and the author from the standpoint of his researches on human voice.

Caruso was also much attracted by the analysis of his own voice, and his vocal apparatus. His own experience and the author's scientific knowledge coöperated in studying him as a vocal phenomenon, trying to find the link that so closely related his art to natural laws.

CHAPTER XVII

THE RADICAL REFORM OF VOICE CULTURE THROUGH THE SPEAKING VOICE

In the suggestions laid down at the beginning of this book for the purpose of reinforcing in actual form the scientific principles of voice production for bringing about a radical reform of voice culture, the following is of prime importance:

Voice culture must be *natural* in its basis, built upon scientific principles; not empiric or arbitrary. There must be only *one* method of singing, founded on physiological laws, taught in a practical form.

This suggestion constitutes the principal basis for the radical reconstruction of voice education as conceived by the author, who emphasizes the speaking voice as the fundamental element for the thorough education of the voice, particularly inasmuch as it is related to the art of singing.

In applying its rules practical evidence is given of the advantages resulting from centering on the speaking voice all the practice required for the training and the development of the voice, either in talking or singing. Thus the marked difference between this method and those existing at present is made evident, from the very beginning.

Making the speaking voice the fundamental element for singing is an issue which has a scientific basis, as has already been demonstrated in this book; therefore, presenting this method of voice culture as "scientific" is not claiming for it an arbitrary qualification; it is a logical outcome, derived from its intrinsic character.

This, however, must not suggest the idea of an artificial method on account of its qualification as scientific. As a matter of fact, the word "scientific" has often been misrepresented by artificial practices; the general impression, therefore, tends toward that misleading belief.

But in the case of the scientific culture of voice, science, which is reinforced principally by rules of physiology, acoustics, and phonology, working in harmonious coöperation, constitutes an essential aid in discovering and estimating at their proper value the functional laws of nature, making of them an illustrative method of voice culture, elementary in its structure and true in its contents.

We therefore emphasize the fact that scientific and natural culture are, in reality, synonymous, in order to satisfy those outside of the scientific field who, from traditional habit, are inclined to balk at anything which bears the stamp of scientific in reference to the human voice. Science is knowledge based on truth, and is very simple in its doctrines. Nothing, in fact, is simpler than the physiology of the vocal apparatus, which conforms with natural laws, and which disregards all theories or statements based on hypotheses or personal impressions, without the support of a scientific demonstration.

While many schools of singing, by making the

art of teaching an elaborated exploitation of exercises better suited to physical culture than to an art essentially emotional and intellectual, expose the students to a strain which often fatally injures their vocal organs, the Scientific culture of voice, keeping very close to the natural mechanism, exploits a simple and elementary method condensed into a few rules. These rules are molded fundamentally on the speaking voice and controlled most essentially by the idea of protecting the vocal apparatus from any strain during the act of singing.

Hence, the aim of directing the art of singing toward a radical reform and of placing it on a firm and scientific basis is made possible by this fundamental change of its culture, in its very roots.

The rules governing this new form of voice culture are summed up in the elementary principle, of establishing proper diction as the basis for a correct singing voice production. This naturally embraces the correct placing and formation of the voice, first in talking, and then its development along the same line in singing.

Although this principle is most essentially related to and is more important for the singing voice, it is applied through the medium of the speaking voice, which, constituting the backbone or skeleton of the singing voice, supplies all its physiological and psychological characteristics— pitch, volume, quality, expression, etc.

The Scientific culture of voice, by developing in detail the author's original view of giving the proper phonetic production to the speaking voice for producing the singing voice with the same mechanism, gives the latter the advantage of finding its words already correctly produced, of molding its volume and quality on that of the speaking voice, and of magnifying its resonance and expression by the addition of its musical colors.

A big and beautiful speaking voice, in reality, furnishes splendid material in the raw for a correspondingly big and beautiful singing voice; the larger amount of musical vibrations and melodious quality of the latter representing merely an acoustic embellishment.

In spite of its importance, very little indeed is known about the proper production of the speaking voice, especially as a phonetic platform for proper singing and voice development.

It is the belief of the author, as the result of many years of study on the mechanism of the voice, and the experience gained through the constant observation and care of many of the greatest singers, that most of the failures in the singing profession are due to the ignorance of the important rôle played by the speaking voice in relation to the art of singing.

The two forms of voice, the speaking and the singing, being the same physical element, are so closely connected that the neglect of one means the abolition of the proper production and beauty of the other. It is no exaggeration to state that the proper formation of the speaking voice is the only *sine qua non* condition of correct singing, as the latter always retains the former's original characteristics, whether beautiful or ugly.

The idea, therefore, of creating a system of teaching which begins by establishing all the rules for the production of a beautiful speaking voice, that the singing voice may be molded on it, has been materialized by the writer in this method, which has been submitted to some of the greatest singers and voice experts.

The recognition of its real value has been expressed to the author in letters and indorsements commending its universal use in voice culture, as can be seen in the testimonial of Enrico Caruso, quoted in a preceding chapter, and those of Emma Calvé, Galli-Curci and Titta Ruffo which follow.

The preface of this book, written by no less an authority than Victor Maurel, the artist who was the first in the musical world to carry out the conception that singing is merely musical speaking, is of the most valuable support for the Scientific Culture of the Voice.

Madame Galli-Curci, in a letter written in English, has given her full endorsement to the principles illustrated by the author, who has also received a very enthusiastic letter from Madame Emma Calvé, translated herewith from the original, which is also reproduced.

A literal translation of the indorsement given by Signor Titta Ruffo for The Scientific Culture of Voice, as conceived by Dr. P. M. Marafioti, follows on the next page.

Endorsement of Madame Emma Calvé for the Scientific Culture of the Voice:

DEAR DOCTOR:

I have just read your admirable book in which you explain with clarity a perfect method in which voice culture must be based on new scientific principles adaptable to the exigencies of the music of to-day. This new method, having become a necessity because of the evolution of the modern school, which demands above all lyrical declamation rather than the "Bel Canto" heretofore required.

Dear doctor, you who through your science have so marvelously known how to fathom the mystery of the voice, you are the one designated for entering into this reform in which you should be encouraged and highly praised.

"The sound soars to the sky," the great poet Baudelaire said. Thanks to you, it will raise us, I hope, to the spheres of eternal harmony—our aim for all.

Your sincere friend,

EMMA CALVÉ.

Endorsement of Titta Ruffo for The Scientific Culture of the Voice:

I have read with keen interest the scientific and practical study on human voice as conceived by you, and found it so marvelous that I feel it my duty to express my opinion in writing.

It will be of great help to all students of singing and declamation because of its extreme clarity and simplicity, which can be seen to perfection in the proceeding by which you develop your new theories. It is necessary that it be given out for publication, so that it may be known in all conservatories of music, and in all schools of singing and declamation.

The education of the voice plays a very important rôle in our intellectual life, as the most elevating emotions of our souls are aroused by the harmony of sounds; and singers as well as actors will be vocally perfect if they learn to abide by the principles which you express in your method.

TITTA RUFFO.

RITZ-CARLTON HOTEL.

MADISON AVENUE & FORTY SIXTH STREET.

NEW YORK

TELEGRAPHIC ADDRESS.
"RIZCARLTON"

UNDER THE DIRECTION & MANAGEMENT OF:-
THE CARLTON AND RITZ HOTELS, LONDON.

1st December 1921

Dear Dr. Marafioti.

I have read your very
interesting manuscript
accompanied by your
kind letter in which
you ask for my opinion.
To my way of thinking
your ideas are not
at all too hazardous.

I find everything
based on scientific
foundations which,
after all, are the only
sound and real ones.
When these exist we
can garnish them as
we desire with art
and sentiment and
give the public the
sweet illusion of

169

FACSIMILE OF MADAME GALLI-CURCI'S ENDORSEMENT OF "THE SCIENTIFIC CULTURE OF THE VOICE"

12 Janvier 1912.

Cher Docteur, je viens de lire votre
admirable livre. J'ai tout expliqué avec
une clarté, une méthode parfaite que
la culture de l'esprit doit être basée sur des
principes scientifiques nouveaux s'adaptant
aux exigences de la musique d'aujourd'hui.
Cette nouvelle orientation étant devenue
une nécessité, à cause de l'évolution de
l'art moderne qui exige surtout
la déclamation lyrique bien plus que
m'en demandait-il tel canto —

170

FACSIMILE OF MADAME CALVÉ'S ENDORSEMENT OF "THE SCIENTIFIC CULTURE OF THE VOICE" (TRANSLATED IN TEXT)

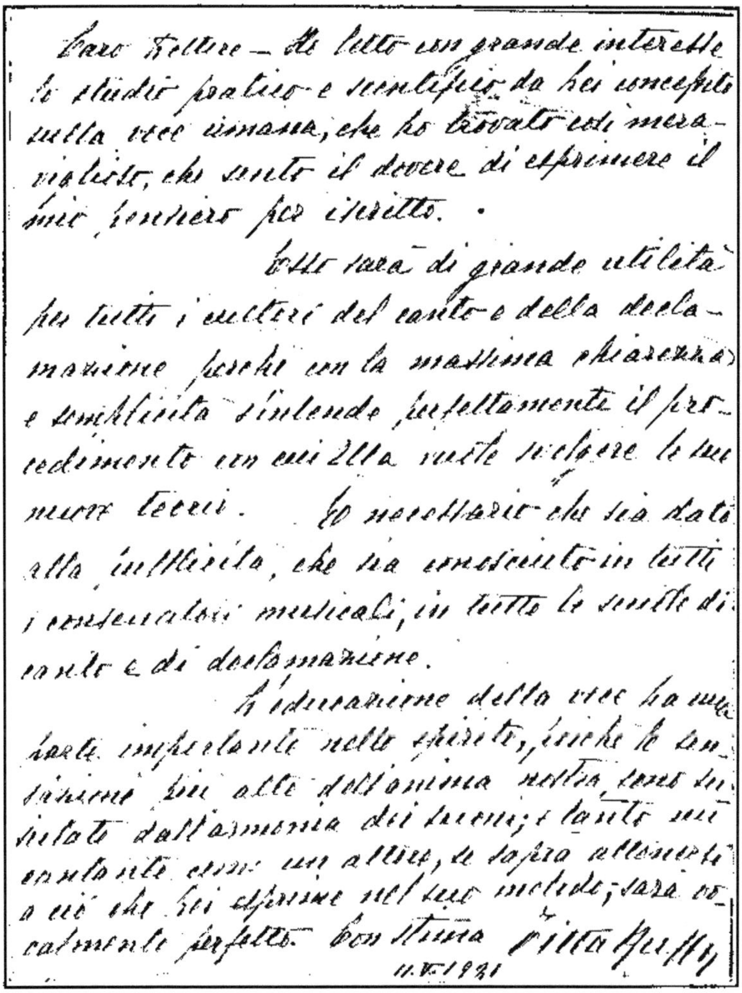

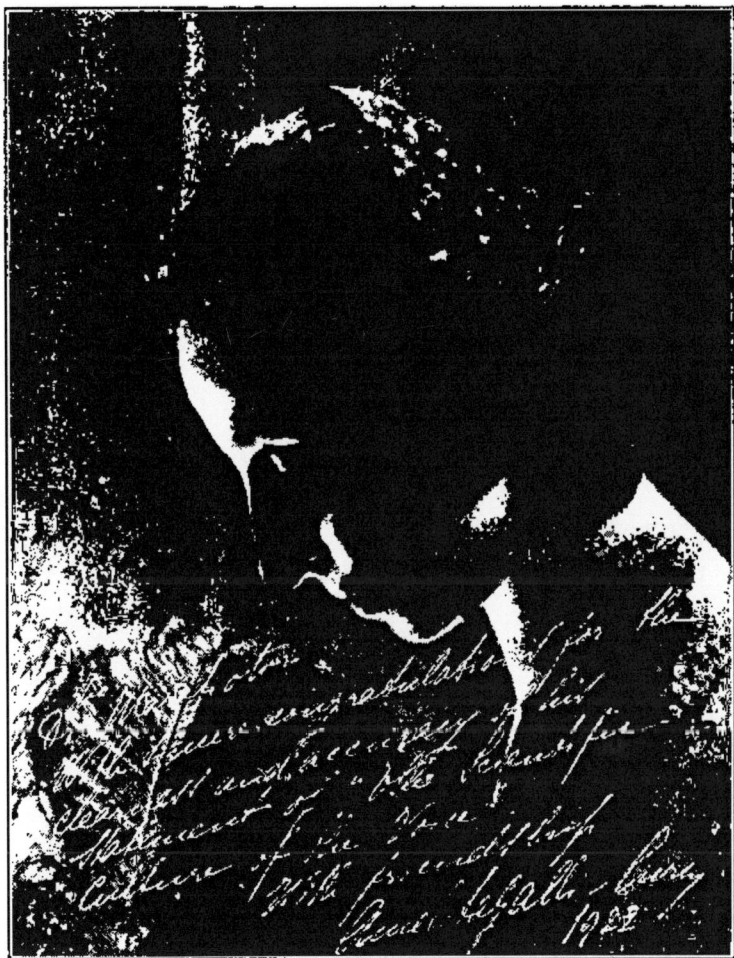

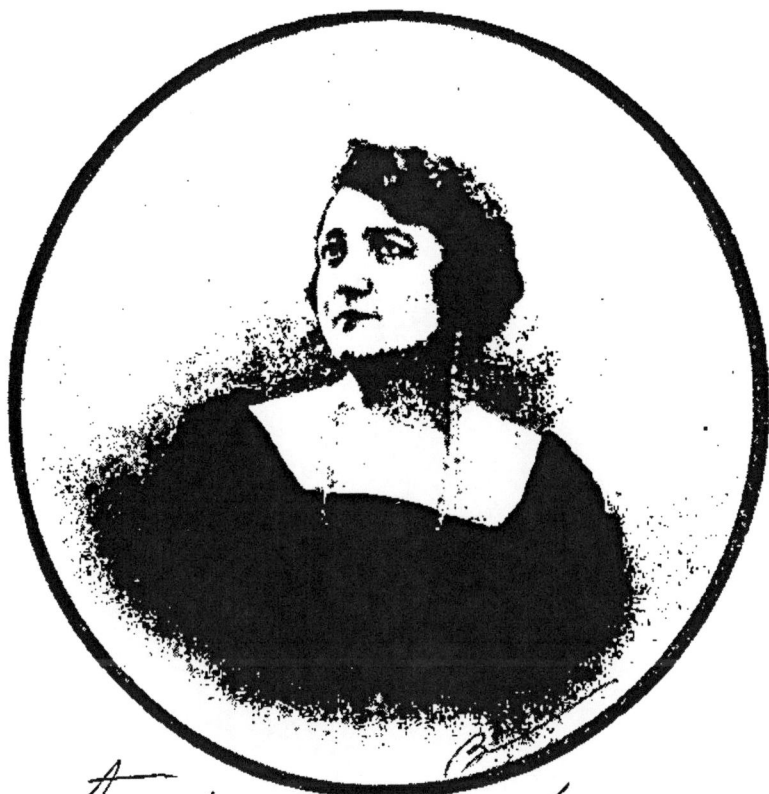

Au savant docteur Marafioti, qui a su démontrer si admirablement la production de la voix humaine. Son admiratrice. Son amie 1922 Emma Calvé.

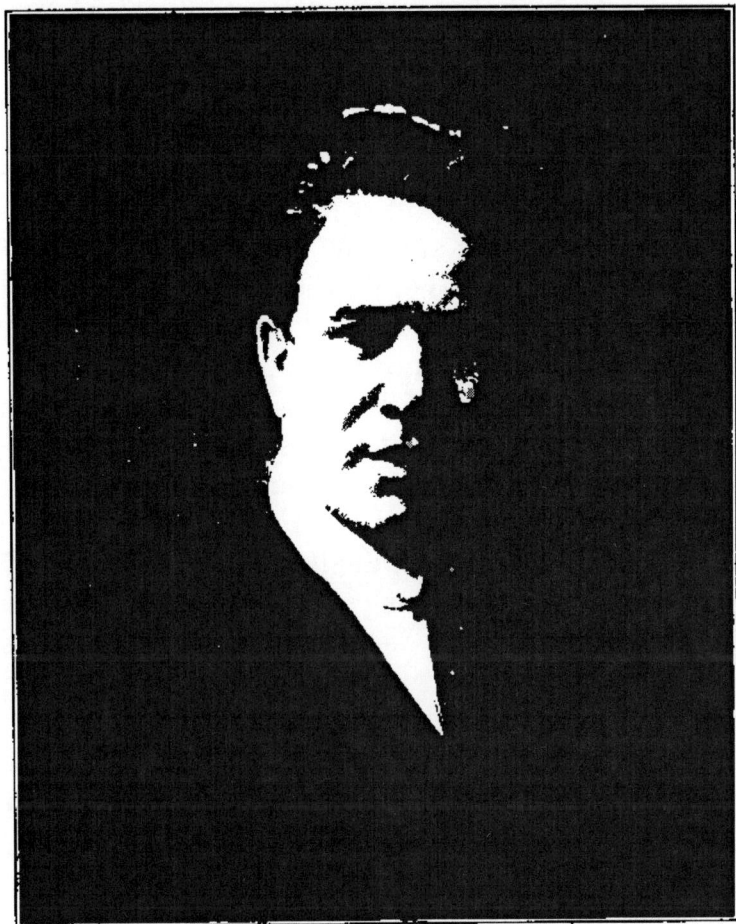

Caro Marafioti — non trovo aggettivi laudativi degni per esprimere tutta la mia ammirazione riguardo i suoi studi scentifici nella ricerca estetica dell'arte del canto, per i quali si dedica con tanto entusiasmo. Con sincero affetto Titta Ruffo

25.X.1920

177

From the *psychological standpoint,* because of its importance, the relationship of the speaking and the singing voice deserves far more attention than is usually given to it. It is not the sound, in fact, produced by the singing voice that gives the impressive power of expression to the art of singing, but what is said and how it is said, through the *medium of tones.* Whether the sentiment the artist wants to express be tragic, dramatic, or lyric, he must have tragedy and drama in his soul, and convey them through his words in order to get a really artistic effect. Intense emotions, in singing, cannot be expressed alone through the medium of tones, tones being rather the medium for musical effects and technical embellishment. They may emphasize an expression which intensely pleases and delights the ear, decorate the singing words in a more beautiful manner, make the phrasing more artistic, but they have not sufficient power to convey a strong message of the mind or an intense pathos of the heart, to an educated audience. If simple tones could do that, there would be no difference between musical instruments and human voice, but indeed nobody can deny that the human voice is the really supreme power and magic medium of human souls, which alone has the privilege of carrying with words all feelings and thoughts, in any definite degree of expression, and shadows of sentiment.

Therefore, if those singers (unfortunately many) who, by blowing very hard, under high pressure of the diaphragm, or whispering softly in their throats with falsetto or head voices, think that they are expressing hate or love, sorrow or delight, they are mistaken. Their psychology is lacking or false, and their singing is very far from reaching the minds and inspiring the souls of any artistic audience. To hear tones which do not carry the impressiveness of the meaning of the words is indeed of very little value to a discriminating public, who wants to know what message the singing conveys.

There are some artists, though, whose singing never fails to reach the hearts of the audience. Among them are a few prominent ones, who combine all the treasures of their voices with the finest sense of expression, and so have the privilege of delivering to the world the most sublime and artistic singing. Everybody, of course, is affected by the beautiful and intense spell of their performance; but not everybody knows of what immense value and support to their artistic efforts is the proper use and intelligent coöperation of their speaking voice. When these artists sing, not one word is lost, and the audiences cry and laugh with them, because they understand them and are carried away by the emotions embodied in the words they are singing. There lies the secret of the striking suggestion and powerful impressiveness of their voices, and this is also what gave its magic power to Caruso's singing.

But how many singers make the audiences understand even in what language they are singing? How many have the slightest notion of this

inestimable coöperating factor—the speaking voice
—and make valuable use of it in their art? Opera-
goers could easily answer this question.

In some recent instances in New York, when
operas were produced in English, there was general dissatisfaction and criticism because not a word
the artists were singing was intelligible to the
audience. If American audiences were more
familiar with the Italian, French, Russian, or German languages, they would soon realize that the
same complaint could be applied to the majority
of singers singing in any language; nay, some allowance must be made for the singing in English,
as this language is, in truth, more difficult in its
enunciation than most of the above-mentioned.
There is an intrinsic phonetic deficiency in the language itself, of which we will treat later.

The lack of discrimination and also of interest
on the part of some audiences about this matter is
responsible for the singers' underestimation of the
importance of singing their words, thus making it
possible to deliver properly the full message of
the music as the composer felt and intended it.
Those audiences, generally, place their interest and
center their enthusiasm only on the top notes of the
sensational singers, and real art means very little
or nothing to them.

The singers, however, or musicians who are attracted by the importance of this subject, should
refer to the following comment by Wagner in
Actors and Singers and see what his conception of
the rôle played by diction in singing was:

"If to-day I seek out singers for a passably correct performance of my own dramatic works, it is not by chance the 'scarcity of voices' that alarms me, but my fear of their having been utterly ruined by a method which excludes all sound pronunciation. As our singers do not articulate properly, neither for the most part do they know the meaning of their speeches, and thus the character of any rôle entrusted to them strikes their minds in none but general hazy outlines, after the manner of certain operatic commonplaces. In their consequent frenzied hunt for something to please, they light at last on stronger tones (*Tonaccente*) strewn here and there, on which they rush with panting breath as best they can, and end by thinking they have sung quite 'dramatically' if they bellow out the phrase's closing note with an emphatic bid for applause.

"Now it has been almost amazing to me, to find how quickly such a singer, with a little talent and good-will, could be freed of his senseless habits if I led him in all brevity to the essentials of his task. My compulsorily simple plan was to make him really and distinctly speak in singing, whilst I brought the lines of musical curvature (*die Linien der Gesangsbewegung*) to his consciousness by getting him to take in one breath, with perfectly even intonation, the calmer, lengthier periods on which he formerly had expended a number of gusty respirations; when this had been well done, I left it to his natural feeling to give the melodic lines their rightful motion, through accent, rise and fall, according to the verbal sense. Here I seemed to observe in the singer the salutary effect of the return of an overwrought emotion in its natural current, as if the reducing of its unnatural and headlong rush to a proper rate of motion had spontaneously restored him to a sense of well being; and a quite definite physiological result of this tranquilization appeared forthwith, namely, the vanishing of that peculiar cramp which drives our singers to the so-called head-note (*Gaumentonn*, lit. 'palatal tone'), that terror of our singing masters, which they attack in vain with every kind of mechanical weapon, although the enemy is but a simple bent to affectation, which takes the singer past resistance when once he thinks he has no longer to speak, but to 'sing,' which means in his belief that he must do it 'finely,' that is, make an exhibition of himself."

The author feels no hesitation nor scruples in affirming that this wonderful statement by Wagner contains more truth and sound precepts about singing than the dozens of books he has read on voice culture. With his accurate analysis of the actual conditions of the singing field, and with a touch of sarcasm and criticism about the operatic commonplaces prevalent among the ordinary singers, Wagner has condensed into these few lines the *most solid, scientific,* and *artistic principles* of the *art of singing.* The real essentials also for correct and artistic singing are so masterly outlined that they make all other methods for voice culture, existing at present, unworthy of comparison.

All the physical and physiological doctrines of teachers who are hunting for sensational phrases and impressive words, the meaning of which is often unfamiliar to them, but serves the purpose of appealing to the unskilled, untaught, enthusiastic pupils who are open to any unknown ideas, become insignificant and ludicrous when compared with the truth condensed in the few suggestions of Wagner in which he leads the singer to the "essentials of his task," making him "really and distinctly speak in singing," and "restoring him to a sense of well being, and to that definite physiological result of tranquilization, namely, the vanishing of that peculiar cramp which drives our singers to the so-called head-note—that terror of our singing masters, which they attack in vain with every kind of mechanical weapon, although the enemy is but a simple bent to affectation, which takes the singer past resistance when once he thinks he has no longer to speak, but to 'sing.' " Much crime—unpunished crime—is committed in the name of physiology and presumably physical theories.

Although Wagner's ideas, in truth, did not influence the author's views in reference to the contents of this book—as the above quoted precious document of the genius of Bayreuth came to our knowledge when this work was almost ready for publication—yet we feel that Wagner's precepts, and the principles on which we base the reform of voice culture, coincide so closely that it is a matter of inestimable pride, as well as invaluable encouragement, to us.

In the author's mind was always imprinted the fundamental principle that *singing* must first be *saying*. If in his creed, which has been inspired by prolonged observation of the decadence of the art of singing and careful investigation into the causes, he has been preceded by such an authority as Wagner, he attributes the greatest of good fortune to this coincidence, and regards Wagner's conception of the art of singing as the strongest endorsement and defense for the reinforcement of his principles.

CHAPTER XVIII

THE VOICE IN ITS RELATIONSHIP TO MUSIC; THE
IMPORTANCE OF THE SPEAKING VOICE IN
VOICE CULTURE

THE essence of the speaking voice, from the physiological standpoint, and its importance as related to the mechanism of voice production either in talking or in singing, has been largely treated at the beginning of this book, especially in the chapters dealing with the principles about the relationship of the speaking and singing voice, and the determination of its pitch and of its dimensions, like quality, volume, etc. (See Chapters XIII and XIV.)

But the importance of the rôle played by the speaking voice, from the *psychological standpoint,* either in dramatic art or as psychological basis for the singing voice, although not an integral part of our program, as previously explained, is a matter of such concern that it is unavoidable to enter for a moment into the field of psychology.

When the primitive man tried to give vent to his first emotion of joy, fear, or astonishment—most probably an indefinite, bewildered sensation —he cried out a sound which constituted the first phonetic expression that vibrated in the air and gave rise to speech. It was a psychological influence which inspired it, and, no doubt, the gigantic impression which struck him—the sight of the sun, perhaps—was the first incentive for compelling him to express his feeling by ejaculating that sound. This constituted the primitive form of language spoken from which speech took origin, having as its inspiration and incitement a psychological sensation striving for expression. Thus it came about that the human voice has been ruled and controlled entirely, from its very beginning, by psychology.

"Le mot, qu'on le sache," said Victor Hugo, "est un être vivant . . . le mot est le verbe, and le verbe est Dieu." "The word, it must be known, is a living being . . . the word is the verb, and the verb is God." Such an important mission has Victor Hugo seen in the word that he compared it to God!

Aside from his poetic emphasis, certainly Victor Hugo was right. There is no medium for expressing human sentiments or feelings so high, so strong, and so effective as to bear comparison with the human voice. Its power of impressiveness is incommensurable, not only in relation to the significance of the words spoken, but at times even independent of them, when it lies wholly and intrinsically in the timbre and inflection of the voice itself. Its sound is the first to strike our ears, and to arouse our interest, which is attracted principally by its color and quality, independent of the contents of the words. That explains why certain great artists—Tommaso Salvini, for instance, or Sarah Bernhardt, or Eleonora Duse, and even the celebrated *diccuse* Yvette Guilbert—conquered the world, often performing for audiences who were not even familiar with their languages, but were deeply affected by the accent, the clarity, the beauty, the pathos, and musical color of the timbre of their voices.

This very characteristic of the human voice exercises a power on us even in ordinary life, to the extent that we sometimes feel repulsion or attraction for a person only because of his voice; sometimes even on account of the sound of his name. Alexander and Napoleon perhaps would not appeal to our imaginations as they do if, instead of their names, they had been called Prosdocimus and Zoroastrus.

Thus it seems obvious that voices having a melodious inflection and beautiful timbre impress us immediately and afford us immense pleasure, regardless of the contents of their speech.

As for the significance of the word, of which the human voice is the supreme medium, its power of effectiveness is far more inestimable than that of the simple sound, which, in spite of its beauty, can never approximate the same effectiveness on human beings as can words.

The infant expresses his first needs and sensations by indefinite, instinctive sounds, which possess little power of impressiveness; but the voice of a baby pronouncing for the first time "ma-ma," or "pa-pa" is a stirring emotion and triumphal feeling well known to all parents.

The effect which a word of sympathy can exert on a distressed soul cannot be equaled by any other psychological or material means. By a word, an entire existence or a destiny can be changed; but, that word, which possesses so much power, does not retain its value unless the manner in which it is delivered carries its full message. Therefore its striking power of convincing and impressing depends principally on *how* it is said, which discloses the great importance of the euphonic enunciation of the speaking voice, not only by itself, but *even more* in connection with the *singing voice.*

Hence the relation of the voice and the music, as it takes place in singing, makes even more conspicuous the necessity of an intimate relationship between the speaking and singing voice, and the standing of the former toward the latter as a fundamental basis for singing.

This relationship is discussed here purely from the *psychological* standpoint, and refers principally to the power of effect of the words in music.

Indeed, music without words has no specific means for expressing love, hate, fear, joy, enthusiasm, admiration, contempt, and all the shadows of human psychology which can be represented and portrayed so profoundly, so exquisitely and so accurately by words alone.

Their great help in making music more effective is made evident by certain celebrated phrases in operas, and even by entire operas. There is no doubt that in the instantaneous and striking success of "Cavalleria Rusticana"—the little masterpiece that conquered the entire world in a few months— a vital part was played by the impressive story of Verga, so beautifully and effectively arranged in libretto form by Targioni-Tozzetti. The imprecation of Santuzza: "A te la mala Pasqua," and the finale: "Hanno ammazato a compare Turiddu," both of which are spoken, constitute two of the most striking and impressive points of the opera, which no doubt swayed the audience to such spontaneous enthusiasm that Cavalleria was marked by immediate and triumphant success unequaled by that of any other opera.

Thus it becomes evident that the words molded into the music can create the most intense and artistic musical expressions, and the coöperation of the meaning of the words with the music is the ideal ground for the growth of the most intense and complete form of art—the singing music. This brings about the logical deduction that, since singing music is strictly dependent on the coöperation of the voice, we must take precautions that this element, of such essential importance, be performed in its highest and most perfect form.

This condition mainly depends on the correct formation of the speaking voice, as the speaking voice in reality lies at the root of the physiological and psychological structure of the singing voice. At its origin, perhaps, the characteristics of the singing voice were first suggested by the speaking voice, which was so beautifully produced as to strike the ears of the listeners with a musical sensation never previously felt, its melodious quality and intonation affecting their emotions in an astonishing manner, and conquering their primitive souls.

The speaking voice, therefore, is the foundation on which the singing voice was built up; and this imposes upon us the necessity of cultivating first the speaking voice as the essential basis for beautiful and correct singing.

CHAPTER XIX

THE CULTURE OF THE SPEAKING VOICE AS THE NATURAL GROUND FOR THE CULTURE OF THE SINGING VOICE

THE physical phenomenon—voice—is, in its simpler and primitive form, originated by a few elementary sounds, which constitute the fundamental pillars of its phonetic structure.

The very roots of the voice are represented by the vowels—five in the classic languages—to which the consonants are attached as complementary elements, thus forming the definite vocal expressions called words. Words constitute the speaking voice.

In developing the culture of the speaking voice in detail, both as a phonetic element and as basis for the singing voice, the author conceived the idea of formulating certain rules, molded on the phonological structure of the Italian language, with the object of creating one sole method of voice culture, of elementary character, easy enough to be understood by everybody and of benefit to students of all nationalities.

This selection is based on the belief that, from the physiological and phonological standpoint in voice production, there is no simpler, more complete, and beautiful language which serves so large a variety of purposes as Italian. Among the reasons which fully justify this preference is the almost universal agreement that Italian is the most melodious and adaptable language for singing; and this statement is not the result of personal opinion, as dozens of books can be quoted, which confirm this assertion and recommend the Italian language for voice training.

Then, too, there is another reason, namely, to establish for voice culture solely one method, with one language as an educational element, which, if universally accepted, would constitute an official standard for voice training. This would materialize the aim of having but one system of voice education for all the singing schools, and would provide the possibility of giving specific principles and rules for vocal training, which, after being recognized as the correct ones, could be applied by the generality, just as all correct principles and rules related to any art or science are universally recognized and practiced. The theory of music, in all its different branches is, in fact, taught and exercised by only one method, with perhaps slight variations, but, on the whole, by substantially the same procedure. Voice education should be the same.

In voice culture, though, voice being the only means for its own training, it is necessary that all the principles or rules which are laid down in regard to its culture be centered fundamentally on the physiological and phonetic mechanism of its elementary form—the speaking voice.

Therefore the phonetic structure of the one language selected on the merits of its phonological elements — vowels and consonants — universally adopted and recognized for teaching, would bring through a standardized technical medium a general understanding on all problems related to voice culture.

It must be understood, however, that these suggestions are intended to serve essentially in assisting beginners and students in their vocal training, or teachers in the practice of their profession. As for singers, after they have acquired the correct vocal technic, through the Italian language, any language should be adaptable and facile for singing, provided they conform their voices to the correct mechanism of voice production.

The author, in fact, in emphasizing the necessity of adopting the Italian language as a basis for voice culture, has no idea of underestimating the importance of other languages, though it is certain that, among the experts on voice, there is much controversy over the relative value of the different languages for singing, while they unanimously agree on the value of the adaptability of Italian.

Dr. Mills, in his book *Voice Production in Speaking and Singing*, says:

"All competent to judge are agreed that Italian, because of the abundance of vowels in its words, is the best language in which to sing, or, at all events, to begin with as training."

Lilli Lehmann in *How to Sing*, writes:

"Without doubt the Italian language with its

wealth of vowels is better adapted for singing than the German language so rich in consonants, or than any other language. The organs of speech and the vocal apparatus, in the Italian language, are less subjected to violent form-modifications. The numerous vowels secure for the singer an easy connection for the sounds, while the poor pronunciation of the many hard consonants interrupts every form—and tone—connection."

As for English, although the author believes that it is not a very flexible language for declamation, nor a melodious, resonant and free one for singing, because of the great number of consonants which prevail in the composition of the words, in comparison with the number of vowels, and the large amount of monosyllables in which the language abounds, yet it is his conviction that most of the deficiency is due to the method of its pronunciation by some English speaking people rather than to the language itself.

As a matter of fact, the manner of speech of the Australians enables them to produce voices that are superior to the English and American in quality and flexibility, and more adaptable for vocal education, as has been proven in the singing field likewise. It is well to remember that Nellie Melba, and a few other singers less conspicuous, have been products of that country; and the author has found from personal experience with some Australian students of singing that there is a certain freedom in the mechanism of their voice production which is dependent on their speaking voice, and is responsible for the pleasing quality they possess, and for their vocal possibilities.

It seems that the scarcity, if not the total absence of English singers in the operatic field is ascribed by some experts principally to the language and its enunciation, though there are other reasons also.

John Hullah, Professor of Vocal Music in Queen's College, gives the following version of this subject in general:

"It is generally admitted that the Anglo-Saxon race, now the majority of the population of Great Britain, are less gifted vocally—have the vocal apparatus naturally in less perfection, and artificially in worse order—than any other variety of Indo-Europeans. As a rule, the English voice, if not always of inferior quality, is almost always, in intensity or capacity, inferior to (for instance) the Italian, the German, or the Welsh. The number of English speakers who can, without too evident effort and for any length of time, fill our largest interiors, or make themselves audible and intelligible at an open-air meeting, is as small as the number of English singers who can hold their own against a modern orchestra, or make their presence felt in every part of the Crystal Palace transept. . . .

"To the foreign and unaccustomed ear the English language sounds, as to the foreign eye the Welsh language looks, made up of consonants, and these hardly distinguishable from one another. As a rule, our speech is wanting both in *resonance* and *distinctness.* We reduce to a *minimum* the *sonority* of our *vowels,* and omit or amalgamate with one another half of our consonants. . . . Certain it is, that from the most sonorous of these—*the Italian* —it is possible to compress into an intelligible sentence many very uncouth vocables, especially when he who uses them knows the value of 'harsh din' as a set-off to euphony."

The most renowned English authority on voice, Dr. Mackenzie, has widely illustrated the value of the Italian language and given his ideas in reference to the English as follows:

"The effect of living out of doors [he says], is not confined to children; one may nearly always recognize a person who spends much of his time *sub dio* by the ringing tones of his voice. Miss Braddon, the distinguished novelist, once told me she has often been struck by the fine voices heard among gamekeepers and huntsmen; and many people must have admired the melodious, far reaching cry of the Newhaven fishwives. I am inclined to attribute the *vocal superiority of the Italians* in some measure to this cause. Every one who has traveled in Italy must have noticed how often trades which in our climate have to be pursued indoors are there carried on in the open air. Tailors, shoemakers, tinsmiths, etc., work *al fresco,* making the streets ring the while with noisy but not unmusical chatter. The balmy atmosphere, as it were, coaxes the mouth to open wide and the demonstrative nature of the people finds natural vent in loud and emphatic utterance. On the other hand, it is a common reproach to Englishmen when they attempt the pronunciation of a foreign tongue that they *will not* or *cannot open their mouths* but make a *rumbling, gurgling* sound in *their throats,* which is presently hissed or sputtered out through the set teeth, as if the speaker were afraid to open his mouth too wide for fear something should get into it. This may be a wise precaution in a climate like ours and Milton apparently attributes our mumbling habit of speech to this cause when he says: 'For we Englishmen farre northerly doe not open our mouthes in the cold air wide enough to grace a southern tongue, but are observed by all nations to speak exceedingly close and inward; so that to smatter Latin with an English mouth is as ill a hearing as law French.' It has also been said to be due to our reserved and undemonstrative nature which leads us to avoid making ourselves conspicuous. Whether this be part of our natural character we must see ourselves as others see us to determine. At any rate, whatever be the amount of our retiring modesty that stays at home, our travelers do contrive (against their will, it may be presumed) to make themselves the observed of all observers wherever they go. And it may be asked, is the climate of Scotland more genial or the character of its people more effusive than ours? Yet Scotchmen have the gift of articulate speech; and display considerable aptitude for acquiring the pronunciation of foreign languages, especially of those in which open vowels predominate.

"Whatever be the cause of our peculiar manner of speaking, there can be no question as to the *utter badness* of it. Nor is there any reason *why this national reproach should continue.* To any one who has been fortunate enough to hear the noble tones of some of our great orators, or the elocution of some (alas too few) of our dramatic artists, the notion that English is an inharmonious tongue may well seem absurd. The music is there, but it needs an instrument to give it voice, and the instrument again must have a player. 'There's the rub.' It is not the vocal organs that are at fault in most cases, but the method of using them. This, as already said, must be taught, and, to be helpful, the teaching must be of the right kind."

The contents of the above quotations are of great value to the author of this book. Although he is not as familiar with the English spoken in England as he is with that spoken in America, he has the impression that the conditions of speech in this country are more deplorable than in the country to which Dr. Mackenzie, Prof. Hullah and others refer.

In certain sections of the United States, in fact, the speaking voice is decidedly deformed by typical, peculiar inflections, and misplaced in its production, being distinctly emphasized in the posterior nasal cavities; while in other sections it is produced much more euphonically, and is more adaptable for drama and singing. The latter sections, however, are exceptional when compared with the English spoken in general throughout the country; but this exception proves that if the pronunciation were phonetically correct, English could be made a singing language as well as most languages, though not to be compared with the Latin languages, which get from the abundance of their vowels and the proper production of their consonants a phonetic mellowness and flexibility which make them almost perfect.

In these languages the case of their phonetic production facilitates their placement in the physiological center of the voice—the mouth—by an almost spontaneous, natural and instinctive act. That is responsible for the smoothness and the melodious characteristics of the Latin languages, which can never be approached by the Anglo-Saxon.

The author has often heard the remark that some great singers—Caruso, for instance, or Galli-Curci, Ruffo, Bonci, etc.—can sing as well in English as in Italian, as far as voice production is concerned. That is true; but their English is substantially Italian in enunciation and accent, the vowels and consonants being placed and produced according to the phonetic rules of the Italian language, and the voice emphasized according to the Italian fashion of singing.

The disparity, in reality, between the Italian language and the English, and more particularly between the Italian and American, lies, at the bottom, in the marked difference in placing and producing the vowels and consonants. By correctly placing and shaping the vowels, and producing the consonants properly, according to the phonetic classification of the classic languages, Italian forms its phonetic elements markedly and distinctly in the mouth. The English-speaking people, on the contrary, particularly the Americans, misplace these elements, giving a decidedly guttural accentuation and tight production. The tension of the laryngeal, pharyngeal and oral organs during the act of utterance is the principal cause. Vowels, when misplaced, become deformed in shape and sound, and by their amalgamation with misplaced consonants produce words which are consequently phonetically deformed, and of disagreeable resonance.

The emphasis given to the act of singing forces these imperfections of voice production to an exaggerated degree, and this marked fault, added to the lack of freedom of the vocal organs, constitutes the essential deficiency of the English language in singing.

In reference to the lack of freedom, and the traditional New England "Yankee twang," Dr. Eugene C. Howe, Professor of Hygiene at Wellesley College, startled his class of girls by declaring that " it is due mostly to laziness of the jaw. It is not attributed to a lack of jaw exercise, but to an unaccountable failure to let the lower jaw fall far enough in articulating."

No doubt the remarks of Dr. Howe have a very strong foundation. Americans are decidedly handicapped in their enunciation by several bad habits, the predominating one of which is talking with their mouths shut and tightened, holding their throats, palates, and especially their tongues, in permanent tension. That brings about a lack of flexibility, because of the stiffness and rigidity of the oral movements during the act of phonation. Americans make of the natural, simple and agreeable act of speaking a very complicated, difficult function. We do not aim to give the impression that we are prejudiced against the American voice production; just the contrary. Our criticism, which is the result of long observation and study on this subject, and is more emphatic than that expressed by many experts on voice, purports to call attention to the real phonetic causes which are responsible for these defects, and to propose a radical reform of them.

It is a fact, regardless of how disagreeable it may appear, that American voice production, with few exceptions, requires much more care and attention to restore it to a natural, easy form of speaking, than is given at present. Americans themselves can scarcely realize how far from natural and easy their voice production is. If they would look at the rigidity of their vocal organs, while talking, especially the throat, the neck and lower jaw, they would be convinced.

This condition is related to many causes: physiological and psychological, but most essentially phonetic. There are some doctors who contend that the climate, dust and noise are responsible for the harshness of this country's voices. Other causes are attributed to a certain psychological influence. Dr. P. Fridenberg, in a booklet entitled *Every-day Causes of Voice Deterioration,* states the following:

"The commoner causes of voice defect and voice deterioration in the average healthy individual may be arranged in three classes, and depend on the climatic conditions, including wind and dust; improper use of the voice, with the factor of strain in loud talking as it is made necessary by our noisy environment, and, finally the lack of attention to voice culture and voice care in our schools. Climate is of great importance for the voice. It is impossible to consider this phase of the subject at length. . . . Another and very important one is the constant noise. In our larger cities it is impossible to keep up a conversation out-doors without unduly raising the voice, and on most car lines it is necessary to shout in order to be heard. In this city the roar of the elevated railways is added, making high pitch and over-exertion inevitable. The amount of effort expended is apparent when we note the facial contortion, the intensity of oral motion, and the loud tone heard during a sudden lull in the street noises. Women are the worst offenders, as they will continue to carry on a conversation at the top of their voices, while most men will, literally, shut up until there is a possibility of being heard without tearing their throats out. American women have been said to converse 'like shrieking canaries,' and this is one of the causes. Another is to be found in the lack of attention to voice and speech in the home and in.the school. In our mixed population, each element contributes some peculiarity or irregularity not only of accent and pronunciation, but of modulation, intonation, and timbre as well. 'Each has some typical defect, and some have a large number. Instead of being corrected at school, the teachers themselves, sprung from the ranks of the immigrant, are like the blind leading the blind. Any one who has listened to the exercises of one of our New York public schools will remember the common, slovenly, and unmusical speech of the average public school teacher. Distinction and precision of speech are often considered affected, even snobbish. It is a fact that nowhere is grace of speech and voice more truly a class distinction than in this country. . . . The great United States language, and especially the variants heard in our large cities, is a marked exception to the rule of clear and agreeable speech. It is true that 'elocution' is taught in our schools, and that there are daily recitation exercises, but little if any heed is given to inculcating the production of beautiful tone, and the precept is nullified by bad example and evil communications which corrupt good speech no less than good manners. The schoolboy imitates the tough and vulgar accents of the street gamin, the college 'man' takes as a pattern the variety actor, the professional athlete and the 'sport' in diction, as well as in intonation. The home is a correcting influence

only in those communities in which there is homogeneity of race, or in the mansions of the wealthy
where English governesses and maids are employed
and the children have a chance to forget the 'American' language."

The author does not fully agree with Dr. Fridenberg on the influence of climate, dust and noise on
the deterioration of American voices. These conditions may exercise a certain influence, but not
one of overwhelming importance, for the same may
be said of other countries and cities, where they do
not exert such a deleterious influence on the speaking voice, nor even on the singing voice. In London
and Paris these conditions are almost the same as
in New York, and the author believes that in
London the voices are somewhat more flexible and
agreeable, and in Paris they are far superior.
Milano has one of the most severe climates in the
world, and is a rather noisy city, yet it is the resi-
dence of most singers and singing students. There
are villages in America with much better climate
and much less noise than New York; yet the
English spoken there is not better, with the exception of some Southern states.

The third reason given by Dr. Fridenberg is,
according to our impression, the most important
one, and personally the author is almost exclusively
concerned about it as the real cause of the deterioration of the American language. It is purely a
psychological influence that is responsible for the

voice production of this country, inherited for the most part, and is the logical result of its phonetic evolution.

It is, as Dr. Fridenberg says, that this country is the out-growth of a mixed population, each element contributing some peculiarity or irregularity of accent, pronunciation, etc., each having some typical defect, and some having a large number.

We all admit that the pioneers of this country, and especially the vast mixed population that came from all Europe, constitute the American masses of to-day, who in influencing even indirectly the American language and manner of speaking, did not lend the most select fashion of speech and pronunciation of their original countries. As the author knows, and as can still be observed among certain Italians, they do not even speak their own national language, but a number of the various dialects. The same condition exists among Irish, Germans, Russians and French of the same class. Therefore, from this *mélange* of common and uneducated voices and pronunciations a pure and euphonic American language could not readily result. On the contrary, the few originally good English-speaking Americans suffered from the influence of the others who infiltrated into the "American" language all the commonplaces of their foreign languages, which they spoke in an inferior and corrupted form.

Thus the American voice production, under these evil influences, was subjected to the gradual deterioration which constitutes, at present, the inherited condition of the deformed American speaking and singing voices. Besides this physical inheritance, is the influence exercised by the homes and schools, as can be observed by following closely a growing child. When he begins to perform the function of speech, under the guidance of Nature, he produces his words with a natural mechanism, in which his vocal organs act without any strain and are ruled by a normal rhythm of movements, under an instinctive rather than an artificial control. Gradually his ears begin to be affected by the voices of the people around, becoming accustomed to forced and harsh sounds. His vocal organs, by the power of imitation, follow the deformed mechanism of his models, until unconsciously he himself falls into the same habits as those who involuntarily influenced him. Commencing from the age of five, six, or seven, his voice changes entirely, and acquires all the characteristics and artificial defects which are prevalent among adults.

The majority of Americans, in truth, make a great effort in talking. They make of the simple, natural function of speaking, which is no different physiologically from the function of eating or breathing, or walking, a complicated performance, in which all the organs concerned work to their utmost efficiency. Yet there is no necessity for contracting the larynx, squeezing the throat, raising the palate, and stiffening the base of the tongue in talking. All of these unnecessary efforts create the sensation of an obstacle in the throat which hinders the free delivery of the speech;

and once that sensation is perceived, instinct suggests a manner of compensating, by augmenting the pressure and amount of breath, which, instead of relieving the strained function of the vocal organs, adds a new element of artificial nature.

The average individual gets accustomed to this mechanism, which establishes the incorrect habit of making *force* the principal element in voice production; and this effort, in the long run, results in impairing the vocal apparatus, adding another cause for disagreeable speaking and defective singing.

In the majority of cases that is the actual fundamental cause of bad voice production, and is responsible also for the lack of expansion, resonance, and ease.

In singing, these deficiencies are the source of innumerable difficulties, particularly since the instinctive conception of singers is to compensate for the lack of resonance with the force of breath—the only help known to them—having been misdirected by singing teachers and by the methods of singing in vogue.

This error, however, cannot be corrected unless we resort to radical means. We must strike at the very origin of these deficiencies, and ascertain the freedom of voice production by the correct physiological and phonetic formation of its very essential elements—the vowels and consonants—and the natural manner of delivering them. This is the most important and fundamental reform to be undertaken; trying to educate pupils to the right conception of the natural function of talking and singing.

Therefore, since English is phonetically rather a difficult language, in some instances made more so by inherited bad habits, we must try to modify it, to smooth it, to produce it in a more natural manner, softening the sounds of the vowels, giving the correct phonetic articulation to the consonants, and, above all, placing both these phonetic elements in the organ suggested by Nature—the mouth.

At any rate, if a reform is to be suggested, it must affect the English phonology as it now stands, and correct it by uprooting it entirely, because that is responsible for the existing conditions.

The materialization of this program must start by giving to children a new phonetic culture, from the very beginning of their education. There would be no practical difficultly in accomplishing this, if public opinion favored this reform. Children learn everything easily.

There are several institutions in America concerned about the necessity of improving the speaking language, but the evil lies in the fact that the promoters are in the awkward position of preaching reforms which they themselves do not practice. In fact, their concern is confined only to the improper inflection of the voice and to the lack of clarity, refinement, and distinction in talking; but as for its correct physiological production with regard to its phonetic elements—vowels and consonants—they are not cognizant of its actual deficiency. If they are, they do not think it of much importance, for they limit all their attention to the English language in itself, without investigating its defects by comparison with the classic languages.

As a matter of fact, it is certain that as long as the vowels are produced in the throat, and the consonants are phonetically misplaced, bringing about a forcible function of the vocal organs, nothing can fundamentally and substantially modify the voice production.

As for singing, the American-spoken English brings about defects which are more difficult to deal with than almost any other language.

There is no exaggeration in stating that Americans, in spite of their natural gift of beautiful voices, which among women are so abundant, and their inexhaustible ambition, are more handicapped in the art of singing than anybody else, and consequently very few good American singers exist, as far as *proper voice production is concerned.* It is true that English in itself is not an easy medium for singing, but with the American pronunciation it is made even more difficult.

While we are aware of the objections that this statement will arouse, we are convinced, nevertheless, that this is actually so.

A natural feeling of protest and a sense of reaction are innate in all mankind. We resent being told our faults. It is an illogical weakness which should not affect educated people, for without criticism there would be no exchange of thoughts nor incentive to progress; yet it does affect individuals as well as communities or nations, often with evident disadvantage.

Therefore, even after statements like those made by Prof. Hullah, Dr. Mackenzie, Milton, etc., about the English and Italian languages, and those of Dr. Mills and Lilli Lehmann in reference to Italian for singing, to which a hundred more could be added, resentment and objections to our view are not unexpected. We think it proper then, to quote an opinion disagreeing for the greater part with ours, so as to let the reader decide impartially which one, in reality, is of greater advantage to American singers. It is our aim to convince people that English, and especially "American-English" is by no means a language fit for voice culture; it must be understood, though, that we do not mean for singing, in its finished form, but only for vocal training. For this purpose we wanted the support of all authorities who are approximately of the same mind. We point out now an opposing view by Leo Kofler, organist of St. Paul's Chapel, New York, and singing teacher also, which is quoted in a book on voice by a foremost American laryngologist, who shares his opinion:

"It is true, as Kofler says, that the Italian language presents few difficulties to the singer. In it pure vowels predominate and consonants are in the minority, and even then many of these consonants are vocal, while the hard aspirates of other languages, especially German and English, are unknown to Italian lips. But that which is easier, by no means is always the most artistic. Ease rarely leads to depth. And this ease of pronunciation may account for a lack of dramatic grandeur and vigor in Italian and for the Italian's method of tonal emphasis and vehemence of gesture.[1]

"The German or the English artist has no need for such extravagances, because the immense richness of these languages—the great variety of vowels and the vigorous aspirated elements—gives to his utterance a dramatic freshness and force which are life and nature itself.[2]

"The English language is probably the one that has been described by foreigners as the most unfit for singing. Greater calumny has never been uttered. I contend for just the opposite; that English is the very best language for an artistic singer to use, for it contains the greatest variety of vocal and aspirate elements, which afford an

---

[1] The fact that "ease of pronunciation may account for the lack of dramatic grandeur and vigor in Italian" makes us think of Tommaso Salvini, the great Italian actor who played not only in Italian repertoire, but also Shakespeare in Italian, for English as well as American audiences. The effects of his artistic voice of which we still hear, were not lacking in dramatic grandeur and vigor, which, on the contrary, were very prominent, despite the fact that he possessed the *easiest pronunciation*.

The pianist, the dancer, the tennis player, or the acrobat, does not lack in grandeur or vigor because of his ease in performing; and the unfortunate horse who pulls a heavy truck along a road littered with stones is not very much pleased with his dramatic grandeur and vigor in accomplishing it. He is trying to go ahead until, obliged to give up for lack of strength, he stretches himself out on the ground. Ease, after all, is not such a deadly evil in the world as Mr. Kofler seems to think.

[2] Lilli Lehmann, the great German prima donna and intelligent artist, in a quotation already given in this chapter, shows that she is of the contrary opinion.

artistic singer the strongest, most natural and expressive means of dramatic reality. The English language has all the pure vowels and vocal consonants of the Italian; and besides, it is full of rich elements, mixed vowels, diphthongs and an army of vigorous aspirates. I admit that it is not as easy for singing as Italian is; but just here its true merit and advantage arise.

"The difficulties thus forced upon the singer compel him to study deeply and perseveringly; but the treasures thus unearthed and placed within his reach will amply repay for hard work." [3]

The views of Mr. Kofler, which leave much room for discussion, have, in recent years, been the predominant concern of certain circles in the musical field of America. A campaign for the worthy purpose of standardizing the "American" language for singing, especially in opera, has been widely patronized by prominent figures in the musical world. Societies have been organized, lectures delivered, opera companies formed, and even all the unsuccessful prima donnas, anxious to seek success in a new field, interviewed. It was unanimously agreed that foreign languages for singing should be ostracized and English imposed. The result was as follows: In some opera houses where all operas were sung in English, most of the audiences openly

---

[3] We can appreciate the true merit of anybody compelled, because of the difficulties of his language, to study it deeply and perseveringly; but we do not see the benefits accruing to voice culture by training the voice through as difficult a medium as the English language, when it can be so easily avoided by adopting a much more convenient one.

declared their dissatisfaction and deserted the houses. "How can anybody," they said, "enjoy a performance of Carmen in English, and one in which it is impossible to understand even what they are singing?"

As for American operas written on English librettos, which have been given by the largest operatic institution in this country for several years, they also brought out evidence of the real sentiment of the public. Their performances were criticized by the critics and the audiences principally on account of the language. Furthermore, in one of these operas it was generally remarked that in the cast which included only one foreign singer, the others being American, this singer was the only one whose words were intelligible to the audience. One could barely detect that the others were singing in English, though when the same artists were called upon to sing in Italian they usually could make themselves better understood.

This proves that there must be some causes related to the voice production of American singers, or to the language in itself, or to both, which become more conspicuous in singing and are responsible for these conditions. The enunciation of American singers, with very few exceptions, is painfully tight and so throaty that only with difficulty can their words reach the audience. Yet it cannot be entirely the fault of the singers. The language, too, is responsible, to a certain extent, as is shown in the case of the foreign singer above mentioned, whose singing was intelligible, certainly not because of his superior intelligence, but rather because he molded his English on a foreign language in which he was trained, and by that means he could sing much easier in English.

It is not unpatriotic to recognize and admit the existence of these inconveniences. It is more so not to try to overcome them. We know of a very prominent American prima donna—an artist more than a prima donna—who has always refused to sing rôles in English. We admire her frankness and courage, though we think that if her voice had been correctly placed and trained at the beginning of her vocal studies by molding it on the Italian language, she would not find English so objectionable for singing, since, with the aid of her exceptional intelligence, she sings in all other languages which do not possess the phonetic difficulties of the English.

Therefore, we claim that English can be made a good language for singing if its training is begun with an easier language which secures the natural placement of the voice and the correct freedom of its production. But we do not agree at all with the opinions emphasized by Mr. Kofler, that English is the very best language for an artistic singer to use. This statement contains an exaggerated dose of praiseworthy but not helpful patriotism.

At any rate it is the general opinion that English is not the best language for singing much less an easy medium for voice training, and that the American-spoken English is not the most pleasing tongue to the ear, as has been remarked most fre-quently by prominent American laryngologists and voice experts. If, therefore, singers, actors, and speakers are handicapped in delivering their voices properly because their vocal organs act under a dif-ficult mechanism, why not resort at the start of their vocal training to an easier language, Italian, for instance? If the formation of the English pho-netic elements is not easy and proper, why not go to the very root of this troublesome cause and apply a radical remedy?

These conditions suggested to the author the idea (which, in truth, is not intended for reforming English phonology, but only for simplifying it in behalf of those who are directed toward a stage career) of giving to beginners and students the phonetic rules of a new language, thus appealing to their imaginations in a new manner which stimu-lates the upbuilding of a new conception of the phonetic mechanism of voice production.

By this means speaking and singing can be per-formed in a natural and easy manner, the voice be-ing placed, with the guidance of another language, in its scientific center—the mouth. Thus singers are enabled to avoid the long and difficult struggle with their vocal organs, which are already accus-tomed to the deformed production of the language they have spoken since their infancy.

A new language is also more apt to train the organs of elocution to radically different adjust-ments, building up an entirely new mechanism. The vocal organs cannot change the habitual rhythm of their function after having worked for years in a certain direction; only a different element, acting under a new influence, can easily readjust it, and for this reason the author feels justified in selecting the Italian language as the most adaptable for this purpose. At any rate, this attempt would not bring any injury to the English, but make it smoother, softer and more suitable for voice culture, and if coming generations gain more possibilities in the field of singing, as a result of the help given to their voice production by Italian as an educational element, the experiment will have been generously repaid, and the aim of the author fully accomplished.[4]

In this method of scientific voice culture, illustrated in the following chapters, the medium adopted for all vocal exercises will be the Italian language.

[4] This conception coincides entirely with the ideas of Wagner, as expressed in the following: "If Italian singing is practicable in a German throat, it can only be through acquisition of the Italian tongue." Wagner, *Actors and Singers*.

CHAPTER XX

BEFORE illustrating the essentials of our vocal method, we wish to make an explicit statement. We do not believe that any method of singing, no matter how simple, clear, and complete it may be, is by itself an efficient medium for voice culture. Students must be taught by competent teachers who alone, through their knowledge and experience, can guarantee that the work of the pupils is correct and progressive. Thus we do believe in teachers, but our belief is conditional.

This method of voice culture has been built on a faithful interpretation of the natural principles which governed the singing of Enrico Caruso, a most valuable example and medium of comparison for students. It will reveal to them how correct, and how close to natural laws our method is, and how to safeguard the physiological rules of voice production advocated in this book. The strongest followers of this method, however, should be the free-minded and unprejudiced singing teachers, those who believe in evolution, in progress, and are earnestly concerned about the restoration of the art of singing. We stated that we believe in teachers, but our belief is conditional; we make reservations about their mission and their methods of practicing the important profession of teaching.

According to our conception, teachers must be the guides and advisers in the solution of the many problems related to voice, and in the application of the natural laws governing it. We do not believe in teachers as creators or builders of voices. There should no longer be room for such charlatans in an epoch in which science controls most of human efficiency and progress.

We do not believe in those instructors who claim that they can benefit pupils by a few weeks of teaching. This is only a commercial exploitation, vastly different from the important profession of teaching the truth about voice culture. As a matter of fact, nobody but Nature can create, make, or build the physiological product of the vocal apparatus—the voice—and nobody can efficiently assist students in their education except by years of constant work in the pursuit of good vocal results, and by mutual understanding.

The art of singing cannot be taught to any one, unless the sense of music, and the call for singing, naturally exist in his soul and blood. To be sure, we owe to nature alone the genius for song. We inherit it with our disposition, enthusiasm, and natural sentiment for singing. The great number of natural singers found among the masses of certain gifted races, who never received any vocal instruction, is the most striking evidence of this. Yet, although a natural gift, our singing may not be correct. The mechanism of voice production, which when correct is the fundamental guarantee not only for good singing, but for the preservation of the vocal organs, may be improperly performed. That is the reason the vocal education must be intrusted to experienced teachers who can insure the proper production of the voice, thus guaranteeing the required resistance of the vocal apparatus for an extended career.

The first duty of the teacher is to ascertain how near to natural is the singing of his pupil, and whether or not he observes the correct rules of voice production. He must then direct the pupil's voice in its full, natural form, through a progressive development, avoiding any attempt to change it by artificial and complicated technicalities.

The singing teacher must keep the beginner's mind free from poisonous theories about the breath support, the artificial division of the voice into registers, and the training of the diaphragm and intercostal muscles (the strength of which must result from years of singing and not from an unnatural development). All these conventional suggestions bear the stamp of scientific doctrines but in reality are banal ideas, opposed to the true physiological rules of voice production. Though they seem important to the elaborate makeup of teaching, in reality they add nothing useful to the learning of pupils, and in many instances prove harmful. The piano teacher does not ask his pupils to familiarize themselves with the physiology of their fingers, nor does he teach them physical maneuvers for developing their muscles. Pupils are not expected to know about doctrines; they must sing by inspiration, free from any artificial influence. The teacher, as a guarantee that his method is correct, must be acquainted with the physiology of the vocal apparatus in general, which calls also for a corresponding knowledge of the anatomy of the vocal organs. It is quite unnecessary for the pupil to know any of this, unless he is interested in making a more profound study of the voice from a scientific point of view. The conventional nomenclature which is so boldly flaunted to impress inexperienced beginners in singing schools is most often founded on arbitrary or imaginary beliefs, and must be condemned. The singing teacher must be thoroughly acquainted with the science of voice for the sake of his pupils, and not merely to make a pompous display or superficial doctrines for vain or commercial purposes.

The singing teacher, capable of judging how near to natural laws is the production of his pupil's voice, will respect its natural production and confine his teaching to a purely guiding influence, leaving the gradual development of the voice to its progressive training. The teacher who aids the pupil in developing his voice, embellishing its quality, extending its range, and perfecting his style of musical phrasing, taking particular care to avoid exaggerated and sensational effects, sets him on the right road for securing a proper and artistic style of singing, thus fulfilling his important mission most efficiently.

When the pupil's voice has certain set faults— either natural or acquired—due to an erroneous voice production, then another responsibility, of more vital importance, is thrust upon the teacher.

The means of correcting voices which have deviated from their natural course, of working on deformed material, deteriorated by incorrect functions of the vocal apparatus, is a problem which schools of teaching have thus far struggled in vain to solve. It is evident that they must resort to different methods.

In reference to this subject there is a perplexing and decisive matter to be settled. Who should be entrusted with the delicate mission of restoring to normal a deformed voice production? To whom, most logically, does it belong; to the laryngologist, to the singing teacher, or to some new professional element? This is the very vital question which must be answered definitely.

"Under present conditions," as Madame Galli-Curci wrote to the author, "singing teachers know very little about the science of voice, and scientists know just as little about the art of singing." That is true. In general the scientific men who are interested in voice are not well enough acquainted with the musical equipment indispensable for the culture of the singing voice; and among the singing teachers very few exist who are at all cognizant of the mechanism of voice production. Therefore, neither of these two elements is eligible to undertake the teaching of voice culture.

The vast number of teachers, whose origin may be traced to that class of singers who, having had short-lived careers because of their bad singing, sought refuge in the teaching field, or those pianists of mediocre ability and no success who tried to commercialize their profession to better advantage, becoming vocal instructors, are not the experienced men to whom the education of the voice can be safely intrusted, especially in its preliminary and fundamental period, which is the most essential in voice culture, and requires a thorough knowledge of the natural principles for its placement and production.

The same objection applies to coaches, conductors, or any other class of musicians (to make no mention of the unscrupulous outsiders of the musical world) who, as a result of failure in their own field, direct their activity to that of teaching singing.

Another prevailing idea in the singing world is that pupils should apply, for their voice education, to the very best singers of the past, or to great conductors. That is a banal error, and a dangerous one.

A child who begins to attend school needs the supervision of an experienced pedagogue to start his education. If, instead, it is intrusted either to a great literary man, or to one who presumes to be such, the child is improperly instructed, for the theories presented to his mentality are not suited to his age. Everybody can see the mistake of the medical student who aims to become a surgeon by assisting a professor of surgery in his operations, without first going through the preliminary studies of anatomy, pathology, and all the other medical branches which are the foundation and support of surgery. In the study of singing, however, this error is casily overlooked. Great artists or conductors are undoubtedly persons well fitted to assist students in their preparatory artistic education for the stage, inasmuch as interpretation and style of singing are concerned. In this they excel all others. But they are not competent in preliminary voice culture, for many obvious reasons.

It is universally known, in fact, that most of the greatest singers never knew how they produced their voices. Prominent examples were Patti, who, as we quoted before, when questioned about her singing would say, "I know nothing about it"; and Destinn, who could explain her physical feeling about her voice, but not her method of singing. Caruso himself tried to investigate his own voice, but his analysis was fruitless. His marvelous singing was natural, eminently natural, and his voice production could not be governed by any conscious influence.

If the great stars who shone in the firmament of opera, and are teaching at present, were capable of forgetting themselves and their artistic achievements, and could teach beginners voice placement and production instead of their own manner of singing, they would perhaps be of more assistance than experience has generally proved them to be. Singing is a personal inspiration and act; no two persons, perhaps, can sing in precisely the same way, though they may have the same method. Two voices, just as two faces, cannot be the same; therefore two mechanisms of voice production can operate along the same lines, but do not produce the same results, and the possibilities of one voice cannot coincide exactly with those of another. The principles are the same, but their application differs slightly, because the vocal means used are different. The majority of great singers of the past sang only by natural disposition and inspiration, knowing little or nothing about the physiology of the voice. As teachers, consequently, they cannot master and apply the physiological laws which are in general unknown to them; thus their instruction must be confined purely to a method of imitation of their own singing, which bears no scientific support. An unconscious self-admiration also seems to be a weak spot in their teaching. Easily enthused with pupils' voices, without judging their personal possibilities at the proper valuation, they try to make them counterparts of their own individuality and art. The result is that most often their teaching proves not only unsuccessful but injurious because it calls for work on too high a mental and physical plane for the minds and voices of the beginners.

We remember a popular and successful lyric soprano, widely known for the beauty of her voice, who owes her downfall to a short course of study with a prominent coloratura star retired from the stage. When the ambitious young singer applied to the great star for assistance to improve some slight shortcomings in her high tones, the teacher felt that in this pupil's voice lay the very chance to reincarnate an edition of herself. Her dream would have been justified had the judgment been correct. The vocal means of the young singer could not withstand the strain of both lyric and coloratura soprano. The teacher, therefore, had to resort to an artificial voice production, which changed the original, natural voice into a series of forced and empty head-tones. The successful young woman went abroad with a voice of rare beauty, which she had used to great advantage for a few years in the large number of simple and artistic songs suitable to her natural means, and returned, after a few months, with the pompous addition to her repertoire of "Casta Diva" and other difficult arias, but not with the same voice of soft, natural, velvety quality, which had formerly made her prominent in the singing field. This artist paid dearly for the tragic influence of her teacher, for she was gradually forced to abandon her public career.

Great artists, it appears, cannot discriminate between their own mental and vocal attainments and those of pupils. They cannot get away from their personal assets, but instead strive to teach their so-called "secrets" to their pupils, in the hopes of making great artists of them. Meanwhile the elementary steps of voice culture are of scarcely any importance to them. Thorough physiological voice production is overlooked in their imaginative and temperamental teaching. It is a lamentable waste of valuable energy, misdirected; it is a regrettable handicap to the progress of the art of singing.

Therefore, who is the man to whom the fundamental education of pupils must be intrusted? The laryngologist?

The teaching of laryngologists endowed with natural musical disposition, upheld by a thorough knowledge of the physiology of voice, could no doubt benefit beginners and singers whose vocal defects are the result of forcible voice production. Since voice is the product of the physiological function of the vocal apparatus, laryngologists, rather than self-appointed teachers, can ascertain if the mechanism of the vocal organs is operating naturally and correctly, and, if not, can restore it to its normal function by detecting the immediate source of these defects and giving the proper assistance to pupils, which the present-day singing teachers cannot. But laryngologists who have sufficient musical experience for competently doing this work are at present very rare. Circumstances are not in their favor. Their professional career does not permit them to cultivate enough music; and the general belief that voice culture must belong only to musicians does not tempt them to enter into the difficult enterprise of restoring to Nature the command of voice production. They could save the present decadence of voice culture, but not without exposing themselves to many humiliations and sacrifices, as their advent into the field of teaching would throw them into competition with professional elements, which, in most cases, are not on equal level with their intelligence, dignity and standing. Hence the men to whom voice culture should be intrusted, provided they acquire more musical competence, are definitely kept out of the field.

To place voice culture in the hands of an infallible element, therefore, we must resort to a new professional man, an expert of the voice, who must combine all the musical requisites indispensable for voice culture with sufficient scientific knowledge to guarantee that singing conforms with natural laws.

This new professional man must be a product of the singing class, selected from those students whose natural gift—voice—is not remarkable enough to raise hopes for a great career as a singer, but whose talents can be utilized to better advantage in the art of teaching. These students, though, must be really intelligent, and endowed with general culture, to be properly equipped to enter a field of this importance.

These students must constitute the professional element which the author points out as the champions for promoting and spreading the radical reform of voice culture, conforming with the principles and suggestions already given. These men must be the founders of that new class of voice experts who will be known as *Voice Specialists*.

The Voice Specialist must possess a keen sense of understanding and of criticism which will enable him to detect the qualities and faults of his pupils. Above all, he must have sound knowledge of the physiology of voice, of its natural production, both as speaking and singing voice. He must be endowed with a fine ear in order to be able to place the voice in its natural center, and take care of its development under the guidance of the fundamental laws of acoustics applied to the vocal apparatus. He must have a facile way of clearly communicating his ideas to the pupil, making himself easily understood, and must mold his teaching according to the plane of his pupil's intelligence. Almost every pupil must be taught in a different manner; the teacher must find the easiest means of impressing his mind with the fundamental needs of a correct method of singing.

The Voice Specialists, although not exceptional singers, must be correct singers, in order to demonstrate to pupils, in practical form, the correct voice production.

To create these new and competent elements, the author advocates a school of Voice Culture for young teachers, which must be founded as part of some important public musical or scientific institution. This school should be recognized by the Government, if the Government feels that this branch of popular education is important enough to be taken into consideration, and if it can foresee of what great service it may be to the musical element of this nation.

Private institutions, private benefactors and many a Maecenas of art are spending millions for the education of gifted young people. Thus far results have been almost entirely negative. Voices exist; ambition, too; money is lavishly expended. What, then, is the actual obstacle?

It lies in the very roots of the elementary education of the speaking voice, from which the real basis of the singing voice takes origin. Therefore, the

Voice Specialists must first be instructed in the correct phonology of the speaking voice.

The method of singing which the author presents in later chapters is merely a continuation of the phonetic method for speaking. If official recognition were given to this method by the Government, starting its application in the elementary schools in the form of phonetic rules, children would learn, from the beginning, an easier and more correct form of speaking. Consequently, those endowed with the natural gift of a beautiful voice would find the road to correct singing an easy one. School teachers should be instructed along these lines, to enable them to competently instruct children.

It is part of the author's program, if aided by public approval and moral support in his attempt to carry out the radical reform of Voice Culture, to establish a special school for conducting the education of those new teachers, the Voice Specialists, who are willing to enter the teaching field through the main door—knowledge and truth.

The Voice Specialists as we suggested at the beginning of this book, must be subject to examination before a special Board of Scientific and Musical Experts, appointed or recognized by the Government. They must get their licenses from this Board, as in the case of any other profession. This alone can protect the singing field from all kinds of intruders, charlatans, and impostors.

This is the aim of the author. The rest depends on public opinion and moral assistance.

CHAPTER XXI

ITALIAN is perhaps the only existing language which has the phonetic property of pronouncing its vowels and consonants always in the same manner. To read Italian it is only necessary to know the enunciation of the twenty-four letters representing its alphabet, all of which take but a few minutes. This constitutes the essential advantage of the Italian language, especially for the student of singing, who, after acquiring a thorough knowledge of the correct pronunciation of the Italian alphabet, finds his voice already naturally placed in its physiological center, Italian being a naturally placed language.

All the phonetic sounds of the English language are included in the twenty-four letters of the Italian alphabet, except the combination of *th* which, however, is very similar to the Italian *d*, pronounced with the breath reinforced a little, while the tongue is held quite relaxed between the teeth.

The vowels, which are the fundamental elements in the formation of the voice, are simpler in the Italian language than in the English, from which they differ greatly, for they are composed of only five sounds, produced very smoothly in the front part of the mouth, while the phonetic organs are kept in relaxation. Therefore, it is of the utmost importance to learn their correct pronunciation, because most of the advantages of Italian, for singing, lie in their phonetic excellence and perfection.

The vowels are five in number, and are always uttered in the same manner, with no exceptions in any case whatsoever.[1] Each vowel has a characteristic shape, dependent upon the adjustments of the organs which take part in its formation.

The first vowel is *A*. It has the sound of A as in the English word *father,* emphasizing its pronunciation in a broad way. It is the largest vowel, and is open and round in shape.

It is most essential to learn the enunciation of this vowel as perfectly as possible, because it represents the first phonetic element from which the other vowels can easily be derived through a simple phonetic evolution.

For its correct production the mouth must be opened wide, though not by a forced movement; the throat, likewise, must be opened entirely. This act should be spontaneous and similar to the opening of the mouth in eating.

To be certain that this important movement is done correctly, two conditions are indispensable: The tongue must lie flat and completely relaxed on the floor of the mouth (see Fig. 19), its

[1] The classification of Italian vowels is similar to that of the Latin and Greek. *See* Goodwin, *Greek Grammar;* Allen and Greenough, *Latin Grammar.*

tip in contact with the lower teeth or lip. The relaxation must be almost passive, no sensation of any sort accompanying the act of pronunciation of this vowel. The palate must be in its normal position, relaxed, taking no part in this phonation.

As very few people pronounce by leaving the phonetic organs in complete relaxation, the author thinks it better for beginners to have these rules more than well emphasized, for they will be of the greatest benefit in singing. To those who have been accustomed for many years to one language, which has very different phonetic rules, it is of great help to exaggerate somewhat the rules of the new language.

It is necessary also to point out that pupils, from the very beginning of their study of this method, must leave aside entirely the English pronunciation in practicing the vowels and consonants, avoiding the confusion of the two languages.

By using only Italian, and always with the correct pronunciation of its phonetic elements, students will acquire the habit of their permanent and proper use.

The vowel E pronounced as in the English words *late, fate,* is but an evolution of the vowel A above mentioned.

In this evolution, the mouth modifies its shape slightly, becoming smaller in size, almost half the size of A. This change is performed essentially outside the mouth, by the upper and lower jaws coming nearer, and making a narrower space in the cavity of the mouth (see Fig. 15).

The organs of phonation—the tongue, palate, etc.—are left in almost the same position as the vowel A, taking very little part in the change, the tongue and palate alone being very slightly raised. The whole difference in the size of this vowel depends on the diminution of the oral cavity resulting from raising the lower jaw toward the upper one.

The vowel I is enunciated like the I in *machine,* and is formed by approaching the lower jaw to the upper one as closely as possible without, however, using any muscular tension. The size of this vowel is the smallest of all. The vocal organs inside the mouth are left in almost the same relaxation as in the preceding vowels, except for a little tension of the tongue and palate, which are raised upward, more than in the vowel E (see Fig. 16).

The focus of the vibrations of the voice in this as well as the other vowels must be centered precisely inside the base of the nose, where a certain vibratory sensation is created and can gradually be felt by the pupil in the form of a tickling sensation, becoming perceptible first in producing the vowel I.

The A, E and I (pronounced as in father, fate, sneeze) are, therefore, differentiated only by the size of the oral cavity, the A having the largest space, the E half the amount of space, and the I the smallest possible without contracting the phonetic organs. The following is an illustration of the comparative size of these vowels, the opening of the mouth to its full extent, without any exaggeration or effort for the A, constituting the starting point in the formation of all of them.

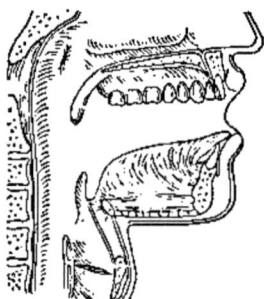

FIG. 14.—THE VOWEL A CORRECTLY
PRODUCED

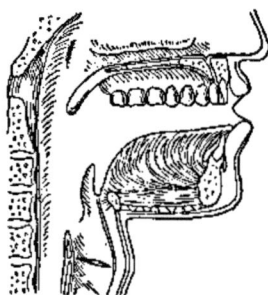

FIG. 15.—THE VOWEL E CORRECTLY
PRODUCED

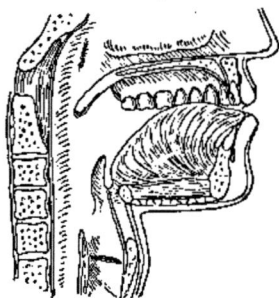

FIG. 16.—THE VOWEL I CORRECTLY
PRODUCED

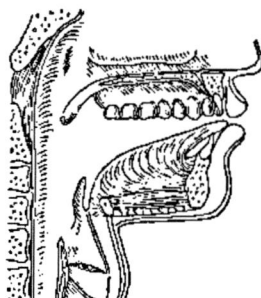

FIG. 17.—THE VOWEL O CORRECTLY
PRODUCED

The vowel O, which has the sound of O as in
bone, is also an evolution of A, in the formation of which the lips play the decisive part by con-
verging into a rounded form, thus closing the
mouth.

Inside the mouth the phonetic organs retain the
same shape during this transition as for A, holding
their same position. This gives O the same space as
A in the mouth, and the approach of the lips forming a megaphone improves the color of its sound,

which gets the characteristic darkness of the O, like a tone produced in a closed box.

The vowel U, pronounced like the U in *prune,* or like *moon,* is an evolution of the O, produced simply by protruding the lips forward, *without squeezing* them, as in the act of whistling or blowing.

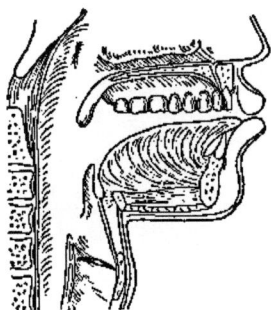

The phonetic organs inside the mouth must be in complete relaxation in the same position as for A, and special care must be taken not to retract the tongue backward in prolonging the sound of the U.

FIG. 18.—THE VOWEL U CORRECTLY PRODUCED

It is of the utmost importance to emphasize time and again that all these sounds must be produced with the complete relaxation of the vocal organs, without any pressure on the part of the respiratory apparatus, with no interference of the laryngeal organs except for the necessary vibrations given to the sound by the vocal cords. In other words, the breath must be normal, the larynx almost passive, the phonetic organs in complete freedom, particularly the tongue. The full sound of the voice must be directed to the mouth, with a specific focus centered in the base of the nose where all vibrations must converge to get the proper resonance.

An X-ray illustration showing the vowels and the position of the tongue during their formation is given in Figures 20 to 24.

The shape of the mouth and the position of the tongue in the formation of the vowels is shown by the following X-ray illustration taken while the vowels A E I O U were being sung by one who took particular care to produce his voice according to the rules of correct vocal mechanism.

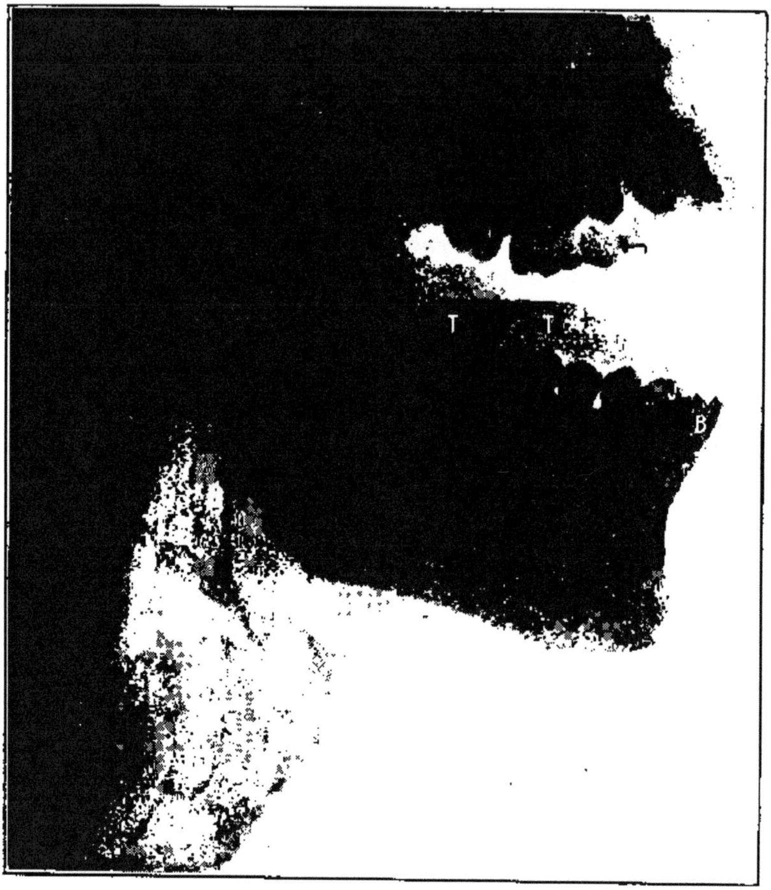

FIG. 20.—VOWEL A

bb. Upper and lower jaw at required distance for shaping a wide-open mouth. *ttt.* Tongue entirely relaxed on the floor of the mouth. The tip of the tongue extends far enough to cover the lower front teeth.

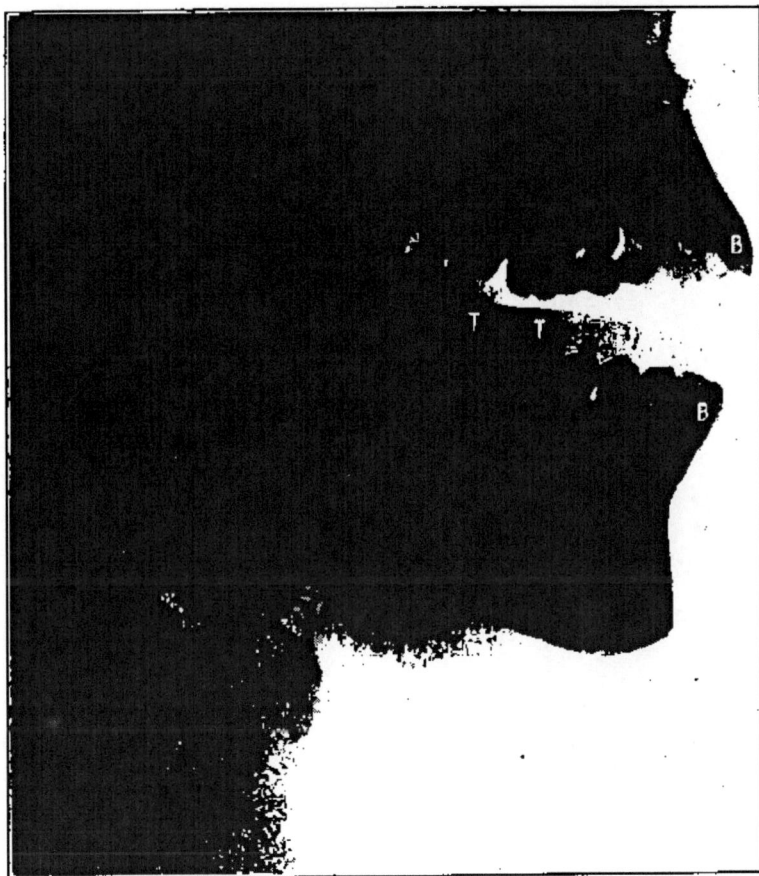

Fig. 21.—Vowel E

bb. The distance between the upper and lower jaw is almost half compared to the opening for the vowel A. This constitutes the difference between these two vowels. *ttt.* The tongue is raised upward only very slightly, but in the same position and relaxation as for the vowel A.

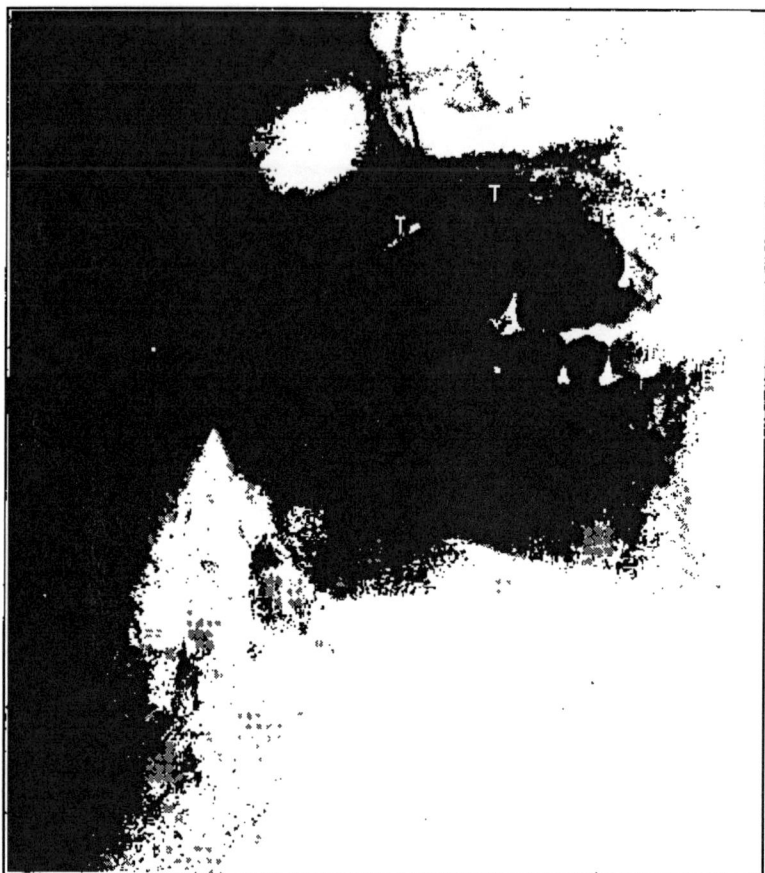

FIG. 22.—VOWEL I

bb. The opening of the mouth is smaller in size compared to the vowels A and E. *ttt.* The tongue is raised upward toward the palate, its tip likewise extending far enough to cover the lower front teeth.

239

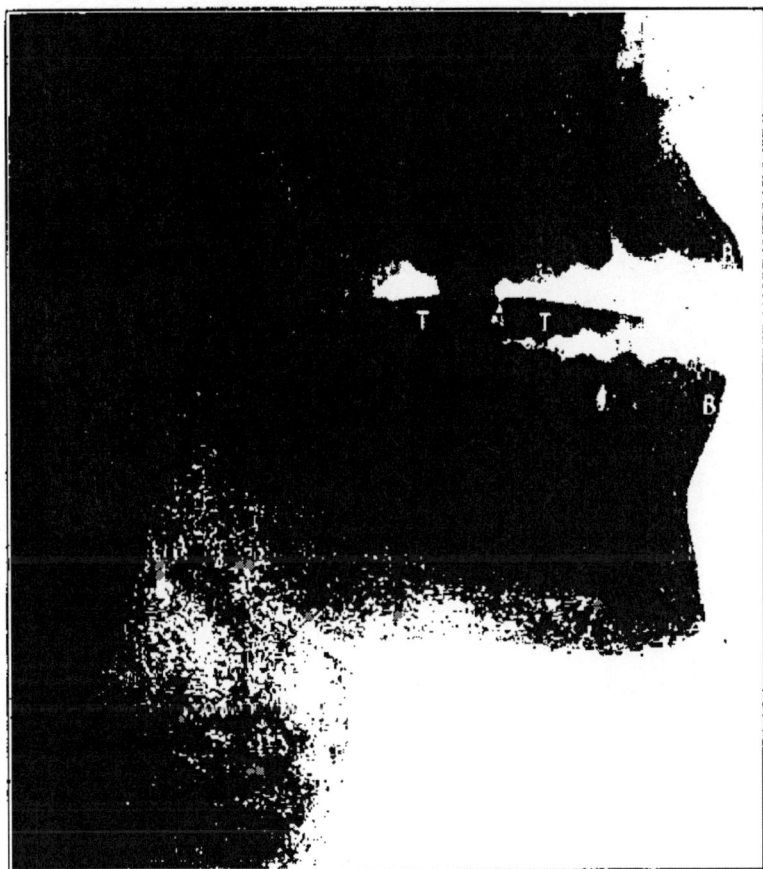

FIG. 23.—VOWEL O

bb. The relationship of the upper and lower jaw is very similar to the vowel A, though somewhat smaller in size. *ttt.* The tongue is in the same relaxation and position. The marked shape of this vowel, is established by the lips, which cannot be seen in the X-Ray,

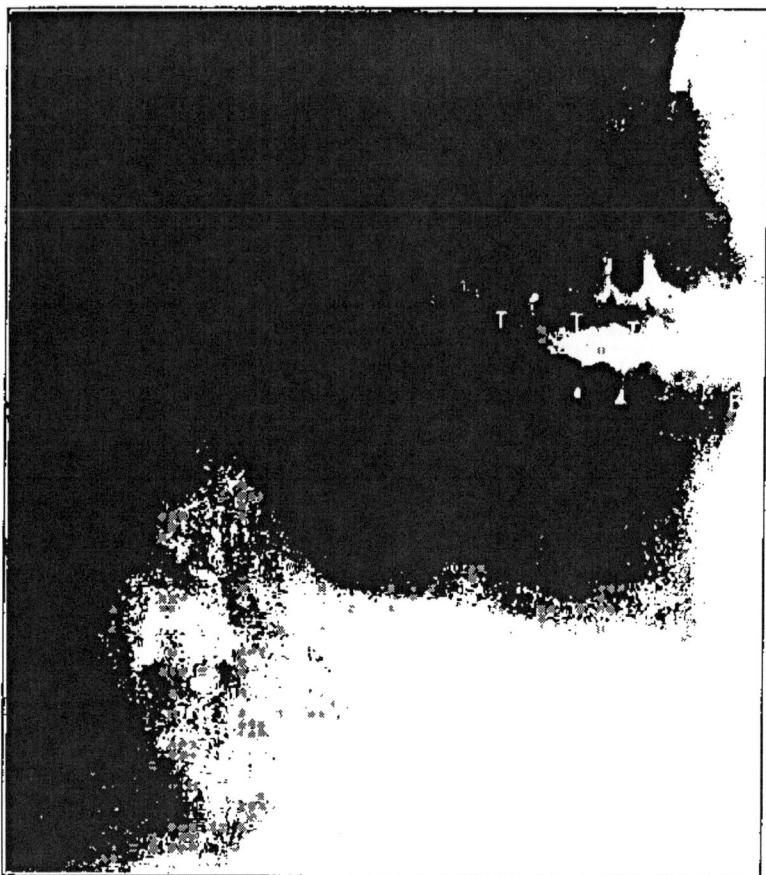

FIG. 24.—THE VOWEL U

bb. The relationship of the upper and lower jaw of this vowel is very similar to the vowel E. *ttt.* The tongue is likewise relaxed and extends over the lower front teeth. The marked difference in the shape of this vowel is established by the protrusion of the lips, which cannot be seen in the X-Ray.

By comparing all the illustrations of the vowels already given in this book with those presented by the majority of books on voice, the readers can see the marked difference in the use of the phonetic organs (especially the tongue and lips) as suggested by this method of voice culture.

Objection may be raised with regard to the accuracy of our suggestions about the pronunciation of the fundamental phonetic elements—the vowels. What entitles us, it may be said, to assert that the pronunciation of the Italian vowels, so different from the English, is the right one?

The answer is a very simple one. Physiologically, their formation corresponds to the fundamental principle of any function, namely, the minimum of energy for the maximum of efficiency. The mechanism of their production, which requires the complete relaxation of the vocal organs, entails no waste of energy. The X-ray illustrations already exhibited show also that phonetically, the Italian vowels are larger in shape, therefore more resonant, more melodious, softer and yet fuller in volume than those of any other modern language.

Hear the Italians talk, hear the street venders calling their wares, and you will realize the most obvious truth.

People who had the opportunity of hearing Caruso, whose voice nobody can deny was the most resonant and full, as well as the most melodious and beautiful, had practical evidence of this statement if only the formation of his vowels ever came to their attention.

The following photographs, taken while Caruso was singing the five vowels, show the different shape of his phonetic organs in the formation of each vowel. On close examination one can almost see the vocal vibrations, running freely all over the masque, and localize the focus of the voice.

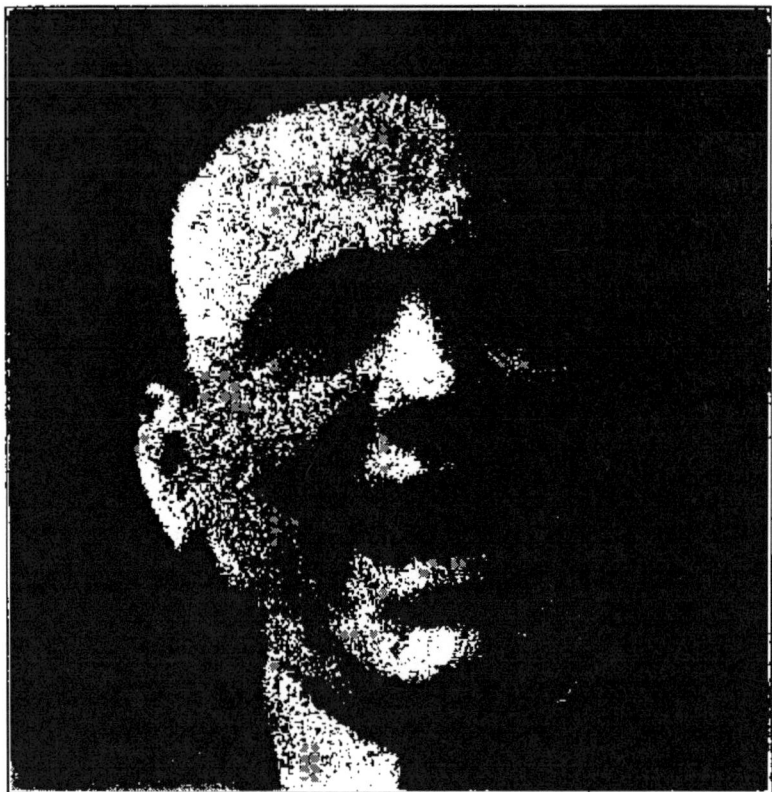

Photo by Bettini Syndicate, Inc.   Fig. 25—VOWEL A

In this illustration the great tenor is singing the vowel A, with very dramatic expression. Note how wide his mouth is open, while his lips are completely relaxed, and his tongue lies flat on the floor of the mouth, its tip in contact with the interior of the lower lip.

243

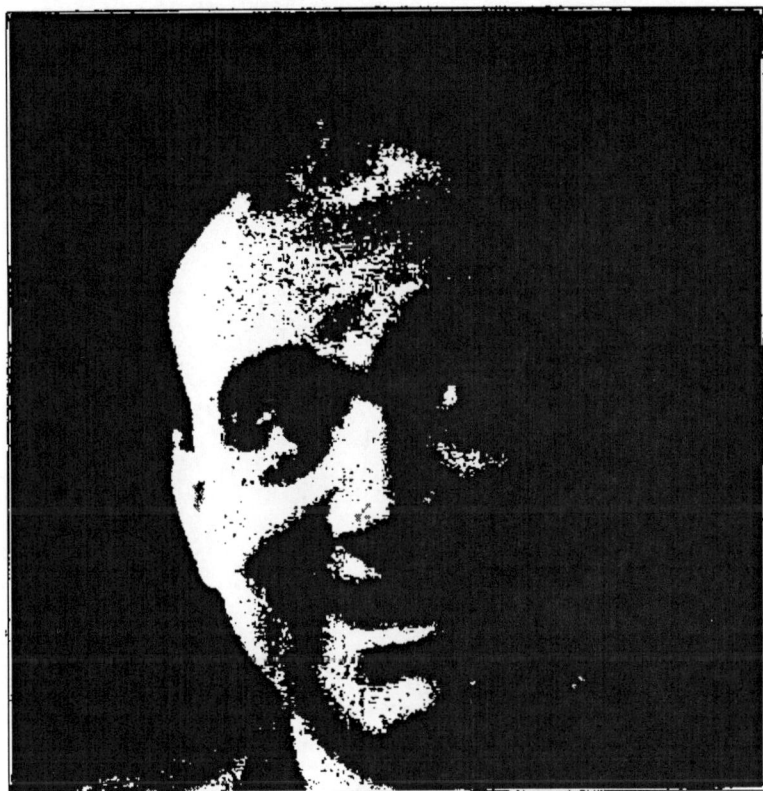

Photo by Bettini Syndicate, Inc.

FIG. 26.—VOWEL E

This illustration shows Caruso singing the vowel E, with lyric expression. The mouth is half open when compared with the size of the vowel A. Note the marked relaxation of the masque and tongue which, as in A, is in contact with the interior of the lower lip.

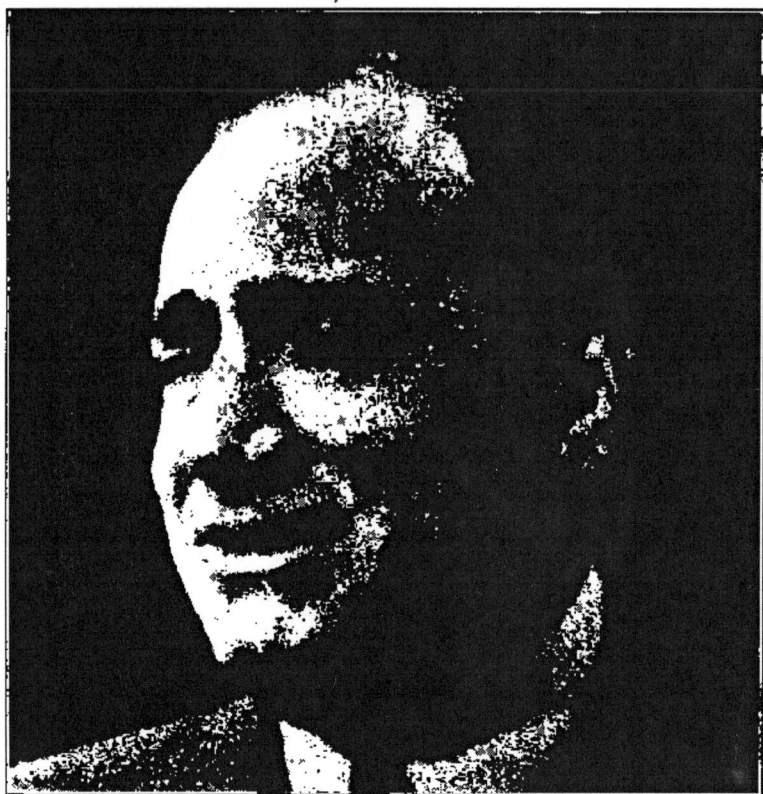

Photo by Bettini Syndicate, Inc.

FIG. 27.—VOWEL I

In this illustration Caruso is seen singing the vowel I. Besides the
relaxation of the masque, as in the vowels A and E, and its characteristic
expression which makes it almost evident where the focus of the voice is
centered, his lips approach without the slightest evidence of tension.

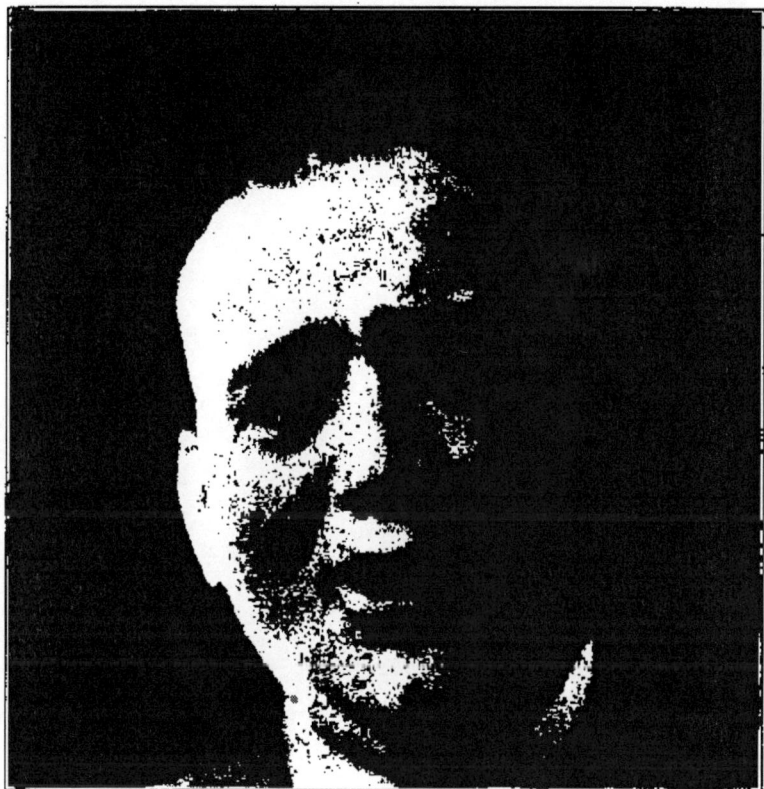

Fig. 28.—Vowel O

This illustration shows Caruso singing the vowel O. The prominent feature lies in the shape of the lips, which are protruded, making a megaphone for the vowel. The lips, however, are in complete relaxation.

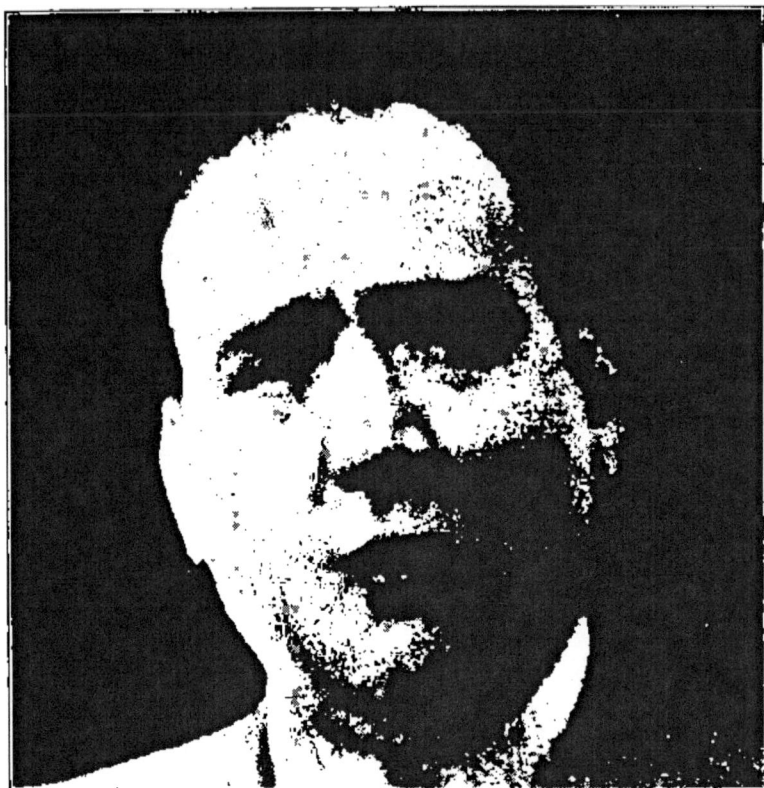

FIG. 29.—VOWEL U

This illustration shows Caruso singing the vowel U. In this vowel the prominent rôle is played by the lips, which by protruding markedly give the shape to the vowel U.

It is otherwise known that Italian is the natural descendant of the classic languages—Latin and Greek—from which it has adopted its phonetic rules. These constitute a most valuable and precious inheritance, and are the best asset in building up its phonology.

All these illustrations reinforce the author's assertion that the Italian language forms its vowels by a correct physiological and phonetic mechanism, and these practical examples given by Caruso justify the broad statement that Italian is the most adaptable and most suitable language for singing.

Although we have already given all the rules for the formation of the Italian vowels, we think that, in practicing, it is advisable for pupils to associate them with the Italian consonants, which, by their articulation, succeed better in placing the voice in its natural center for singing. As a matter of fact, it is true that the sound of the voice is given by the vowels,[2] but phonetically its placement is more distinctly directed by the consonants. Their denomination of Labials, Linguals, Palatins, etc., serves to indicate the place where they are to be articulated, and the organs which take part in their production. The consonants, therefore, are of great help in the correct pronunciation of the vowels, and a sure guide for the placement of the voice.

[2] The word vowel, in fact, is derived from the Latin *vocalis*, the root of which, *vox, vocis*, means voice. Therefore, vowel means voice.

CHAPTER XXII

ITALIAN molded the formation of its consonants entirely on the Latin language. This accounts for their correctness which, even independently of other reasons, is confirmed by their natural, easy production.

The consonants of the English language, on the contrary, are the very phonetic elements which have greatly deteriorated from their original pronunciation in the classic languages, and do not conform entirely with the natural laws of voice production.

The phonetic rules of the classic languages established certain classifications of the consonants, based on the predominant use of the organs taking a prominent part in their formation, which have not been retained by the Anglo-Saxon languages, except in a small part. This has brought about differences in the mechanism of the vocal organs when producing them, and it clearly shows the causes of their deformity when compared with their original models.

It would take too long to make a detailed comparison between the actual formation of the English consonants, so different from Greek or Latin, and therefore from Italian; but readers who are particularly interested in this important subject may refer to numerous books on voice where the consonants are treated at length in their English form, and then consult any Greek or Latin grammar to ascertain the difference.

The Italian consonants are classified as follows: Labials (lips), Linguals (tongue), Dentals (teeth), Sibilants (whistling), Palatins (palate), and Gutturals (throat. See Figs. 30-31).

Other classifications, with slight differences exist, but for our purpose these will serve best.

The denomination of labials calls for a prevailing use of the lips in pronouncing these consonants, and a specific placement of the voice on the lips. Their exact pronunciation is: Em (E pronounced as in empty), Bi (I pronounced as in machine), Pi, Ef, Vi (pronounced similarly).

These consonants, formed principally by the lips, must be produced only by approaching and putting them in contact without any muscular contraction or pressure. The act must be natural, and without force. This is of the greatest importance in singing, because a production forced even in the slightest degree in talking is always emphasized to a much greater degree in singing.

The pronunciation of the consonants alone, however, is not very important for this method, as they are never disassociated from the vowels in talking or in singing. Therefore, it is preferable for students to become acquainted with their sounds when connected with vowels in forming words, which in voice production constitute the real sounds of the voice.

By associating the labials, M, B, P, F, V, with the five vowels, the following syllables result: (*Read with Italian pronunciation. All exercises should be read from left to right.*)

Ma	Me	Mi	Mo	Mu
Ba	Be	Bi	Bo	Bu
Pa	Pe	Pi	Po	Pu
Fa	Fe	Fi	Fo	Fu
Va	Ve	Vi	Vo	Vu

The ordinary difficulties arising in the pronunciation of these syllables are the following: First, the contracting and squeezing of the lips (especially for the P) forcing the consonants' production, because of the English classification of them as explosives B and P, aspirates F and V, and resonant M, which require a very efficient mechanism, while in Italian no emphasis of the sort is necessary, it being sufficient for their formation to approach the lips and to enunciate them with the slightest amount of breath, taking care at the same time that the organs inside of the mouth take no part in the act of their formation.

Another usual difficulty is to avoid making double vowels during the utterance of these syllables. Many people, in saying Ma, are unconsciously induced to pronounce Maaaa; in saying

LABIALS
M·B·P·F·V

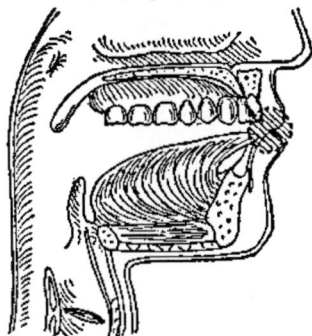

LINGUALS
L·N·R

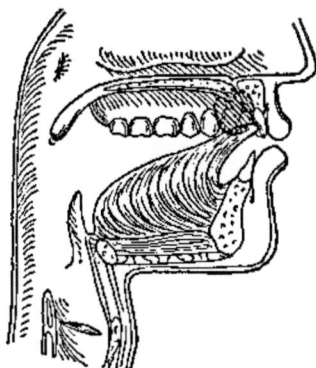

DENTALS
T·D

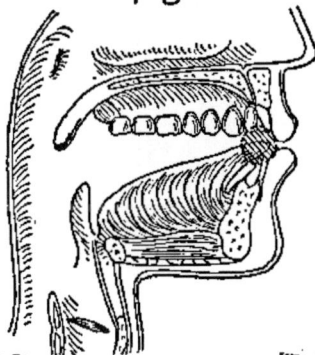

SIBILANTS
S·Z

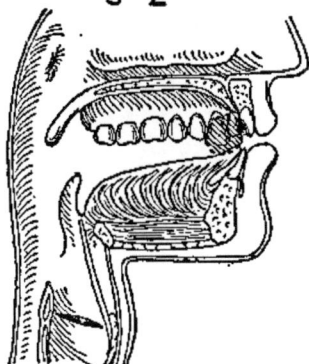

PALATINES
C·G

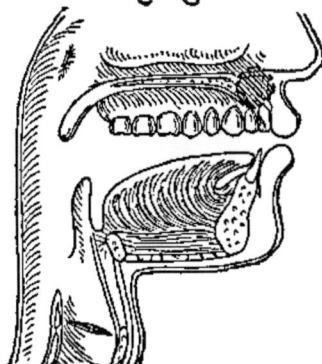

Fig. 30.—Correct articulation of the consonants in accordance
with the classic languages

LABIALS
M-B-P-F-V

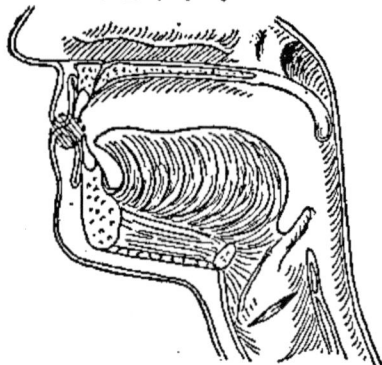

LINGUALS
L-N-R

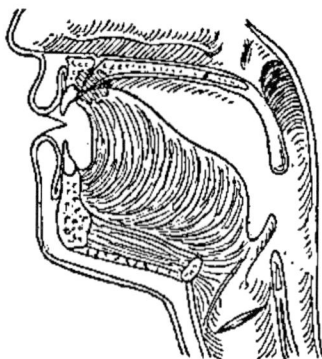

DENTALS
T-D

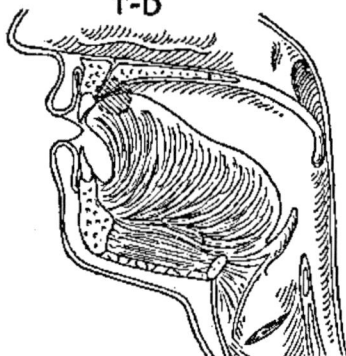

SIBILANTS
S-Z

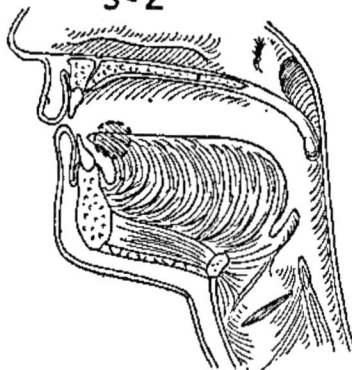

PALATINES
C-G

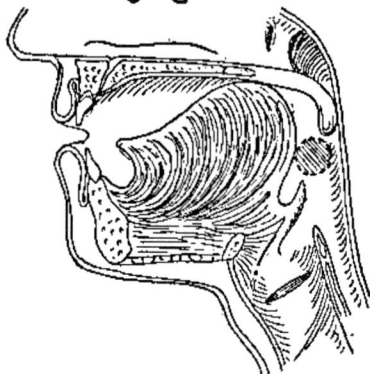

Fig. 31.—Incorrect articulation of the consonants

Me, to pronounce Meeee; Mi, Miiii, etc. That happens because, in prolonging the pronunciation of these syllables, they drag the sound of the vowels by pulling their tongue back toward the throat, accomplishing actually the same act as in swallowing. They swallow their voices.

That can be avoided by reading staccato, and pronouncing only one vowel, like Ma, Me, Mi, Mo, Mu, leaving the *tongue relaxed all the time,* and in contact with the lower teeth.

Likewise particular pains must be taken with their correct formation in reference to their shape, opening the mouth and throat wide for the Ma, and changing its size for the other syllables, according to the rules already given.

The second set of consonants—the Linguals, N, L, R—call for special attention in the use of the tongue for their formation. In English these consonants differ radically from the Italian, being produced by raising the tongue against the palate with a stiff movement, while in Italian the tongue is in complete relaxation, its tip moving very gently toward the upper teeth. Their pronunciation is En, El, Er, the tongue *relaxed* touching the base of the upper teeth. Of the three consonants the most difficult is the R, requiring particular care in the relaxation of the tongue, and its movement, which must be exactly the same as in N. The palate takes no part in the formation of these consonants.

For our purpose it is better to associate these consonants with the vowels, as has been done with the labials. The pronunciation must be in staccato form, avoiding the dragging of the vowels into the throat.

Na	Ne	Ni	No	Nu
La	Le	Li	Lo	Lu
Ra	Re	Ri	Ro	Ru

The usual interferences to be overcome are the stiffening and raising of the tongue against the palate, the double vowels, the forcing of the articulation.

The third set of consonants—the dentals, D, T —are also much different from the English, as they are formed by leaving the tongue between the teeth and pressing it very gently, while in English the tongue is raised toward the front palate, exerting a certain pressure against it. Their pronunciation is Ti, Di, the T produced by using a little more pressure of the teeth on the tongue than the D, which is softer and quite similar to the English *Th*.

In their connection with vowels they are:

Ta	Te	Ti	To	Tu
Da	De	Di	Do	Du

Care must be taken to prevent the same interferences as in the labials and linguals, especially not to stiffen the tongue or force their articulation.

The sibilants, S, Z, differ from the English inasmuch as the English, in their articulation, hold the tongue in tension, and the amount of breath employed is exaggerated.[1] In Italian, the tongue is left in complete relaxation on the floor of the mouth, and the amount of breath used is the smallest necessary. The sound of the S is sweet, and similar to the English C, as in Cinderella, the Z being a little stronger, almost the same as in the English word zuzu.

By relaxing the tongue, and by using a moderate amount of breath, it is easy to get the right sound of:

Sa	Se	Si	So	Su
Za	Ze	Zi	Zo	Zu

The same care must be taken as in the preceding paragraphs not to create double vowels, especially for the *Su and Zu,* which most often are unconsciously pronounced Suuu, and Zuuu, swallowing the *U.*

The palatins, C, G, present more difficulties than the others, as in English they are articulated in the throat with a guttural production in which the base of the tongue and the palate undergo a marked contraction, the breath being forced also. In Italian the pronunciation is approximately that of K, as in kerosene, keen, kalendar; and G is like that in gallant, gospel.[2] The contraction of the

[1] Dr. Mills says that S cannot be sounded without more or less of a hissing sound, suggesting the escape of air, which is very unpleasant to the ear; and unfortunately these hissing sounds are very common in English, so that the speaker or singer is called upon to use all his art to overcome this disagreeable effect.

[2] These consonants, when associated with the vowels *e* and *i,* keep the sound of k only if written with an h between, as in *che, chi ghe ghi.* Otherwise this sound is soft, as in chest, gem, chill, gin.

throat, palate and tongue, and the pressure of the breath must be entirely abolished, leaving the tongue relaxed on the floor of the mouth, the center of the palate slightly raised, and the vibrations of these consonants precisely focused inside the base of the nose.

Singers who succeed in forming these consonants in their natural place establish a wonderful guide for their voice production, as this little center represents exactly the focus of a physiologically and phonetically correctly produced voice. Madame Galli-Curci very appropriately calls it *il puntino*—the little point—and claims that it is the control of her voice placement. When she feels the vibrations of her voice in that *puntino,* she knows that the production is right.

Pupils, especially those endowed with light voices—coloratura and lyric—must try to create some vocalizes by using the consonant C, correctly produced, in connection with the vowels, pronouncing as in Ka, Ke, Ki, Ko, Ku. They will find this the greatest help for their voice placement and the flexibility of their voices.

The guttural consonant in Italian is Q. It is used so seldom that it is not worth devoting any time to it. Its pronunciation is like in English.

Summing up, we see that the mechanism of the formation of most Italian consonants, as compared with the English, is radically different, and the difference lies first in their placement and the mechanism of their formation.

The Italian followed the classification and the

phonetic rules of the classic languages, while the English modified and altered them, with evident deterioration from the point of view of euphony. That deformity brought out the necessity of forcing the mechanism of their production, establishing a false ground for the entire voice production, which is based on the pressure of the breath. This condition, of course, has been of detrimental influence in singing (see Figs. 30, 31).

Pupils, therefore, must attach the greatest importance to the correct formation of the consonants, which in connection with the vowels constitute the corner stone of correct and beautiful talking and singing.

To make it easier for pupils to practice properly the Italian vowels and consonants, the following exercises are arranged in such a way that to the syllables formed by the five vowels and a consonant, for instance *M* in Ma, Me, Mi, Mo, Mu, there is a corresponding syllable attached, made up of *N* and the five vowels in succession, that is, Na, Ne, Ni, No, Nu.

Applying this to the labials, M, B, P, F, V, we have the following:

Ma'na	Me'ne	Mi'ni	Mo'no	Mu'nu
Ba'na	Be'ne	Bi'ni	Bo'no	Bu'nu
Pa'na	Pe'ne	Pi'ni	Po'no	Pu'nu
Fa'na, etc.				
Va'na, etc.				

Linguals, N, L, R.

Na'na	Ne'ne	Ni'ni	No'no	Nu'nu
La'na	Le'ne	Li'ni	Lo'no	Lu'nu
Ra'na, etc.				

Dentals, T, D.

Ta'na	Te'ne	Ti'ni	To'no	Tu'nu
Da'na	De'ne	Di'ni	Do'no	Du'nu

Sibilants, S, Z.

Sa'na	Se'ne	Si'ni	So'no	Su'nu
Za'na	Ze'ne	Zi'ni	Zo'no	Zu'nu

Palatins, C, G (pronounce c like k).

Ca'na	etc.,	etc.
Ga'na	etc.,	etc.

From this first exercise the pupil will gradually pass to the very important one which has the purpose of creating for the vowels alone the same pronunciation as they have when associated with the consonants.

The exercise is:

Man	An	A
Men	En	E
Min	In	I
Mon	On	O
Mun	Un	U

A	E	I	O	U

Ban	An	A
Ben	En	E
Bin	In	I
Bon	On	O
Bun	Un	U

A	E	I	O	U

The same combination of vowels with all the other consonants must be repeated in succession.

In this exercise, when the vowels are pronounced *alone,* particular care must be taken to keep exactly the same formation as in their association with the consonants. The vocal organs must be used with the same mechanism, without emphasizing the breath, without making double vowels, and by giving each vowel its exact shape. Pupils are usually inclined to pronounce as follows: Man—an—aaa, Men—en—eee, etc., which is very unsatisfactory, because it can never lead to the correct formation of the most important vowel, the A.

All the above exercises are of great importance, for those same syllables will form the words, or the raw material, which will afterwards be transferred into the method of singing for preliminary training.

By establishing the Italian phonetic rules with the aim of creating a correct and easy medium for voice production in talking, we have founded the most important factor for voice culture in singing. These same rules, brought into the field of singing by the speaking voice, will furnish to the singing voice its proper, natural placement and its correct voice production; above all it will relieve the singing voice of the responsibility of elaborating every physiological and phonetic function related to voice production.

The pupil who will give due importance to the correct formation of his vowels and consonants, and will learn them to perfection, will gain years of profit without struggling with tone production, breathing exercises, and voice building.

CHAPTER XXIII

THE first singers of past ages knew nothing
about singing methods. Instinct suggested that
they embellish their speaking voices with musical
colors and rhythms, thus originating the primitive
forms of singing, ruled by individual methods.
These methods were merely the spontaneous outcome of natural inspiration, sentiment and emotion, musically expressed according to the singers'
intelligence.

A vocal method, therefore, which aims to build
up a *natural* form of singing, must have at its command pupils who possess, in addition to an adaptable speaking voice, the required inspiration, sentiment and intelligence; and it must be applied
individually also, though molded on general fundamental principles alike for all singers.

The aim of this method is to guarantee that the
natural equipment, the voice, is trained and developed according to the dictates of Nature, so that
it will improve instead of deteriorating from its
original form and beauty. As for the inspiration,
sentiment, and intelligence, Nature alone can be-

stow these on pupils. Teachers, however, can direct and develop the psychological dispositions of pupils with advice based on their own experience.

The speaking voice—the primary element for singing—is the basis for voice culture in this method, which in its principles does not differ from any other method for musical instruments.

A close examination of the modern teaching of piano, violin, etc., makes it evident that freedom and ease are the indispensable requisites for a thorough and correct technique. No physical exercises are recommended for strengthening the fingers of a violinist or pianist; it is understood that they will gradually develop their power by long training. Therefore, students of singing, contrary to the general practice, will not be requested by this method to undergo any physical or breathing exercises for putting the vocal organs in readiness for voice culture.

This new point of view about the breath may surprise the majority of readers, but it is our conception that through the normal function of singing, which requires a specific amount of breath, the vocal organs gradually develop, by constant use, enough resistance for any emergency that may arise in the vocal training of pupils. In professional singing, of course, there is some slight difference in the use of breath, as it frequently occurs that a stronger amount of it is required for certain intense musical phrases of operas of dramatic character; but these emergencies concern only finished singers who, after long study and practice, have their voices in readiness for any emergency. Beginners have no right to attempt trials which, in reality, are a danger to even the vocal organs of advanced and well trained singers. Sensational outbursts are very commonplace among inexperienced and enthusiastic students; but these temperamental pupils should recall the fate of Icarus who tried to fly with artificial wings of wax, which melted when he flew too near the sun, so that he fell into the sea and was drowned. Furthermore, they must remember that the vocal organs of professional singers who, on occasion, indulge in strenuous efforts, are physically hardened from long training, while the same effort on the part of beginners brings on fatigue, and paves the way for more disastrous consequences.

Therefore, beginners must start their course of study as real beginners, proceeding in voice culture as they would in learning a new language, art or science. From the most elementary and simple exercises they must gradually advance to more difficult ones, never losing sight, however, of the basic principle, that ease and freedom are the basis of voice production.

Ease and freedom must be psychological as well as physical, each depending so closely on the other as to make it difficult to ascertain which is the actual support in their coöperative mission.

A singer who is positive that he can rely on the full control of his voice and on the normal efficiency of his vocal organs gets from this assurance the strongest assistance in singing—confidence and courage. Hence his physical freedom, the result of his correct mechanism of voice production, becomes the support of his mental freedom which, relieved of the worry of safely getting through the difficult passages, helps to make his singing technically perfect. Thus his mind is concentrated on the meaning of the words, which lends to his singing impressiveness and style.

But in the absence of the support of correct voice production, the singer feels under a nervous strain which destroys his mental and physical freedom. It is true, however, that some singers, by natural disposition, are so affected by outside influences, especially by that inexplicable sensation of stage fright, that they lose complete control of their voices. In some cases this abnormal psychological state of mind influences even singers of renown and renders them entirely helpless, though they can otherwise fully rely on their voices. Good singers, however, may overcome such conditions by long training and will power; but in cases in which the absence of confidence is due to lack of correct voice production, no improvement can be hoped for, unless a new method of singing, the correct one, is adopted.

What is the correct method of singing?

The method of voice production which borrows from the speaking voice the physiological and psychological elements essential to the art of singing, that is, the voice in its physical form, the pathos, expression, clearness, and meaning of its words, and combines them with musical rhythms, colors, and artistic style, is the correct method of singing.

The Scientific Culture of Voice takes its starting point from this conception; thus it begins where the phonetic rules for talking end, without, however, causing any breach, as the culture of the singing voice is but a continuation of the speaking voice's proper formation.

Three conditions are practically indispensable for achieving correct singing.

1. The amount of breath employed must be proportional to the exact number of vibrations required by the tones to be produced; balanced in distribution, and under steady control.

2. The vocal apparatus must act normally, as in talking, with no strain or abrupt adjustments of its organs.

3. The resonating apparatus, made up of all the cavities of the body, must be easily accessible to the vibrations, and must not be hampered in its free distribution of the sounding waves during their expansion.

The first and second conditions are essential in the production of sounds, but the resonating apparatus is the power which lends to the voice its volume, quality, beauty, and all its psychological characteristics; therefore, it is the most valuable coefficient in singing.

In a very sensible criticism, made by E. W. Myer, about the vocal-effort school, as he calls it, and the relaxed school, he very strongly condemns, on one hand, the muscular school which makes of man a mere machine instead of a living, emotional, thinking soul, and, on the other, he makes some interesting comments on complete relaxation in singing. He says that "flexible firmness without rigidity, vitalized position, and action is the only condition for singing, and that the tone of the relaxation school lacks vitality."

We agree on the whole with this statement of E. W. Myer, but we discriminate between the conditions ruling the singing of finished singers, and the essentials needed for voice culture of beginners. In voice culture we discard entirely all emotional influence during the preliminary work of students, in which the full relaxation of the vocal organs is indispensable for properly placing the voice and establishing a correct mechanism for singing. The training of beginners, at least for the first year, must be confined to the simplest form of musical expression, exempt from any strong psychological influence. This period of time is no specific; it is related to the intelligence of the pupils, and their conscientiousness in studying.

The correct phonetic use of the voice and its most accurate mechanism in regard to its placement and production must be the only aim on which they must concentrate their minds and work. This represents the first period of voice culture, in which singing must have the form of musical talking, avoiding all sustained tones and musical effects. When the thorough technique—natural, not artificial technique—is attained, so that a free, natural voice production is assured, then pupils can gradually be led into exercises and practices of more marked musical and psychological character. The "flexible firmness and vitalized action" claimed by E. W. Myer can at this period be gradually employed.

Therefore, the principle we advocate for beginners is the complete relaxation of the vocal organs, leaving the flexible firmness and vitalized action to finished singers who are entitled, by reason of their competence, to make use of all the technical dexterity for embellishing their voices and their style of singing.

The first condition for correct singing, as we stated before, is related to the amount of breath used and its distribution.

The proper amount of breath cannot be mathematically established; if it were possible it would perhaps solve the most perplexing problem of correct voice production. The author, however, believes that as long as its quantity is fully sufficient for the support of the voice, the less breath used, the better the singing. There are two reasons for this:

1. The minimum of breath places the voice on its exact pitch, producing only as many vibrations as are required for a determined note, and not more. The vogue of screaming which prevails at present is principally dependent on the large amount of breath singers use, under strong pressure. The surplus of air is instinctively augmented in the ascending altitudes of the scale, producing very sharp

tones, and establishing that mechanism, so universal nowadays, which makes of most singers strenuous, sharp-pitched blowers.

2. The minimum of breath establishes also a balanced function for all the other vocal organs, besides the lungs, which take part in voice production, that is, those forming the voice—the vocal cords, larynx, and mouth—and those providing its resonance—the body cavities. Therefore, the efficient coöperation of the breath, the throat, the mouth and the resonance cavities is primarily governed by the balanced power of the breath.

At the beginning of the training, in order to produce the singing voice the same amount of breath must be used as in speaking the syllables or words of the exercises. For instance, if the exercise is made up of the syllables Ma, Me, Mi, Mo, Mu, or La, Le, Li, Lo, Lu, the same amount of breath used for pronouncing them distinctly must be used also for singing them. To carry this out correctly the tones must be sung in staccato rhythm, which has the advantage of freeing the vocal organs by using them in rapid adjustments, not allowing them enough time to become rigid. Singing staccato helps likewise to place the voice, for when the syllables to be sung are first spoken correctly, in staccato rhythm, they can easily be kept in the same place for singing. The singer then has no chance to drag the voice backward into the throat, as he often does in singing sustained tones. At times when even the attack of the tone is correct, prolonging the sound of the vowel toward the end makes it throaty. A great soprano used to call this "swallowing the little tails of the vowels."

When the vocal organs begin to operate in complete freedom, and pupils are thoroughly accustomed to the correct distribution of a normal quantity of breath, then sustained tones must enter into the vocal training, as there is no longer danger of a forced production.

Pupils, we repeat again, must not forget that it is not the quantity and power of breath that is of great importance in making voices big and beautiful. It is, rather, its intelligent and balanced distribution, combined with freedom in singing, and, above all, with the largest amount of resonance possible. They must begin their training with the conception that singing is nothing more than musical speech.

The posture of their bodies, therefore, must be natural, as in talking, without artificial maneuvers, just assuming the same attitude as in addressing some one. That helps in getting psychological freedom also.

The vowels and consonants being the fundamental elements of the singing voice, correct voice production is dependent principally on their proper formation.

Just as in a pearl necklace the rarity of its pearls, their size, shape, smoothness, luster, and arrangement make the necklace beautiful and valuable, so in the human voice the perfection of the elements of which it is composed—vowels and consonants— by their clear enunciation, their volume, resonance, quality, and smoothness, lay the ground for perfect and artistic singing. Therefore, pupils must practice very accurately the phonetic rules already given for the speaking voice, and take infinite pains with their production. Associating the vowels with the labial consonants, at the beginning, helps to make the voice placement easier and more precise, the labials being articulated by the lips.

For pupils to whom the pronunciation of the phonetic elements proves an easy matter, it is a good scheme to try, in the first exercises, to associate all the vowels with the consonant L, which though more difficult to articulate, and having a tendency to stiffen the tongue in its production, creates on the contrary a marked flexibility of that muscle when correctly produced.

The flexibility of the tongue is of most essential importance in voice production, as this organ is decidedly the worst enemy of singers, often constituting the most obstinate impediment to the freedom of their voices. By an instinctive act they usually retract the tongue toward the throat, and keep it in tension, thus preventing the laryngeal sounds from freely coming out and reaching the mouth. This causes a serious interference, which must be overcome at any cost at the beginning of voice training, for the flexibility of the tongue assures the freedom of voice production. Demosthenes, the greatest orator of Ancient Greece, thought the tongue such an important organ for the voice that he used to practice his orations with a pebble in his mouth to make his tongue more relaxed and flexible.

It is certain that in the singing of Caruso one of the actual causes of the ease and brilliant enunciation of his voice was the flexibility of his tongue. It was his servant, and without constraint he could shape it in any way he pleased. His marvelous rendition of the "Tarantella" of Rossini was the most striking evidence. One of his peculiarities was his morning inspection of his vocal cords, which he could easily examine by keeping his tongue so flat on the floor of his mouth as to make it possible to see his larynx in the laryngoscope without protruding his tongue, a maneuver which is very difficult even when performed by a laryngologist.

Before a performance the author often saw him pull his tongue repeatedly, to make it more relaxed. By natural instinct he put great faith in the flexibility of this organ, and trained it so well that as a "stunt" he used to hold the center of his tongue concave, and curl the end and side up, forming a cup, triangular in shape.

The tongue, in singing, must be kept in relaxation on the floor of the mouth, except in the production of the vowel I, in which it must be raised slightly, though in relaxation, toward the palate, and in the lingual consonants N, L, R, in which its movement is indispensable for their formation (see illustration of tongue X-ray, Fig. 27).

This method of singing, built up on the speaking

voice, calls also for a demonstration of the use of two other important phonetic organs—the palate and the lips.

The palate, which when naturally conformed and well arched, improves the resonance of the voice remarkably by creating a larger space in the mouth, must be in relaxation also. Exception is made during the enunciation of the vowels A, O. U, in which the soft palate raises the uvula but very slightly, while the tongue is left entirely flat or concave on the floor of the mouth, thus creating the largest space possible. Space in the mouth proves a great coefficient for the volume, softness and darkness of the voice, owing to the magnified resonance.

The lips must always be left in normal relaxation, as in talking. They are of great importance in the formation of the vowels O and U, for, by approaching them without squeezing, a tube is formed in front of the mouth which acts as a megaphone for their resonance, making these vowels soft, dark in quality, and larger in volume.

The attention to teachers and beginners is called to another important matter in regard to the section of the range which must be used at the beginning of vocal training.

The author believes it is a necessity to confine the preliminary exercises to the lowest tones of the range, beginning at the altitude of B or C below the staff, and descending to its lowest part, until the voice gradually disappears. In the case of a soprano or tenor, if the tones are not forced this takes place at approximately E below the staff.

That voice production should commence in the lowest section of the range is advisable for at least two reasons:

1. In the low tones it is easy for pupils to employ the normal amount of breath required to place their voices on the exact natural pitch, while in the higher tones it is more difficult to control this amount, owing to a psychological influence which suggests to singers, in general, to give more breath than is necessary in ascending to the high sections of the range.

2. It is important also to develop the voice (always without forcing), first in its very low part, which, although not used later in singing, for physiological reasons forms the support of the higher section of the range. It has been demonstrated in the first part of this book that the lower the level of the voice, the higher its range can develop; the more correctly the vocal organs produce the lower tones (that means without forcing), the further can the upper range be extended, without effort.

It is similar to the construction of a building. The deeper the foundation, the higher the building. In voice production this proves to be the case, because, having trained the vocal organs to the maximum of relaxation and freedom through the lower tones, by keeping the same mechanism of voice production all through the range, pupils can find no difficulty in producing the tones at the altitude intended by natural laws. As a rule, only artificial interferences make the range of the voice shorter;

therefore, the common belief that Nature creates *short voices* is erroneous.   Short voices are the result of false mechanisms of voice production.

Pupils, at the beginning of their training, must not expect to produce big tones.   Their attention and care must be concentrated only in having their vocal organs operate in complete relaxation, and placing the voice in its correct center, guided by the speaking voice, which, if correctly produced, can establish both the place and pitch of the singing voice.

This new conception of determining the pitch of the singing voice by that of the speaking voice is of the greatest assistance in producing the voice, especially in high tones.   It is a fact that if pupils hear the tone they are to sing, produced by the piano, and succeed in saying the syllable in that pitch, or if by mental influence they direct the pitch of their singing to the altitude designated by the speaking voice, the resulting tone will be easy in production and correct in pitch.   In the first part of this book, in the chapter related to the pitch of the voice (p. 123), this subject is amply illustrated. Beginners and singers should, therefore, learn to talk in any pitch, consequently enabling them to mold every tone of their singing on the pitch of the speaking voice.   The advantages are manifold.

A habit common to beginners, and also to singers, is that of neglecting to open the mouth sufficiently when it is essential, as, for instance, in the vowel A, or of opening it forcibly.   Some teachers object to the opening of the mouth.   It is an error.   The mouth is the door of the voice; it must be opened to allow it to escape. Even instinct suggests that the mouth be opened in producing the voice. When a child starts to cry, which is a primitive psychological expression, he opens his mouth wide. In singing this must be done naturally; not forcibly. In eating we open our mouth spontaneously and instinctively by dropping the lower jaw; the same must be done in opening the mouth for singing, thus avoiding a rigid, muscular mechanism.

In the case of professional singers who wish to learn and practice this method, we caution them that the task is *much more difficult* than for real beginners. Singers, undertaking this, must forget and renounce entirely their previous method of singing; they must put themselves in the place of beginners, which is usually very difficult to do. The more primitive an element they will become, the more will the progressive influence of this method, by gradually substituting new rules for voice production, destroy their originally faulty mechanism. Their practicing at the beginning must be colorless, and more like musical speech. This is very important, because the mere suggestion that they are singing will unconsciously bring them back to their original faults.

It will also be difficult for them to discard the influence of the diaphragm and breath pressure; therefore, it is a good policy for them to remain seated while performing their exercises, as if they were merely talking to the teacher. In this manner they will be kept away form the unconscious psychological influence of their professional singing.

Fundamental voice production at the beginning must be correct, not artistic. Gradually, after the pressure of the breath is controlled, the voice correctly placed, and freedom in singing is acquired, exercises of more musical style can be attempted, beginning with sustained tones in the lower part of the range. This constitutes the second phase of their new training. In the third phase, when this method of practicing the exercises is applied to songs or operas, they have nothing to fear, as their solid preliminary training will have prepared their voices for any vocal emergency.

With these general hints for correct voice production, we have prepared the ground for our vocal exercises.

Care must be taken that they are strictly and constantly observed, if progress is desired. Until pupils get the proper mechanism of voice production they must think of nothing else, nor be influenced by any other ambition. Later they will realize the value of these suggestions.

CHAPTER XXIV

VOCAL EXERCISES OF THE SCIENTIFIC CULTURE OF VOICE

THE pupil, either standing in a natural pose, or seated comfortably, avoiding all muscular rigidity, must conduct himself as if carrying on a conversation.

In the case of professional singers who can hardly overcome the habitual pose of the stage, it is better to be seated, with head bowed slightly, concentrating their mental attitude on the idea of telling rather than singing their exercises to the teacher.

The first series of exercises are staccato in rhythm, and are made up of the five Italian vowels in combination with the consonants B and M in alternation with L, as in Ba, Be, Bi, Bo, Bu, and La, Le, Li, Lo, Lu (Italian pronunciation).

In cases where the pupil finds that another consonant is easier to articulate, he can use it for a preliminary length of time.

It is understood that these syllables must be pronounced very distinctly, observing strictly the phonetic rules of Italian vowels and consonants as given in Chapter XVIII, and special care must be taken to avoid the formation of double vowels.

Pupils, after hearing the exercises on the piano, must first enunciate clearly the syllables to be sung, as nearly as possible on the pitch of the tones played; then, by using the same mechanism as in the speaking voice, that is, the same pronunciation and amount of breath, carry them into singing.

For practical convenience in practicing, we emphasize again, in a brief summary, what pupils must do in singing these exercises, according to this method, and what they must avoid:

1. They must act as real beginners, children, in fact, and they will learn much more quickly.

2. Give no emphasis to what they are singing, except in regard to its correct pronunciation.

3. Have the mental suggestion of being tired; it helps to relax.

4. Open the mouth wide by *dropping,* not forcing, the lower jaw in producing the first syllable, Ma, La, or Ba, etc. The larger the space of the *A,* the greater the resonance.

5. Sing with full voice, not falsetto. Often pupils who are self-conscious fail to give their full voices. This must be avoided, at any cost from the very beginning.

6. Practice before a mirror so as to be certain that the rules are observed. Do not depend on the ear for that; its control can be easily misleading.

7. Watch the tongue; that is of most vital importance. Keep it in soft contact with the lower lip; it helps its relaxation.

8. Sing the exercises in staccato rhythm for three or four months, or more, until the voice is placed

and produced with the vocal organs in complete relaxation.

What pupils must *avoid* in singing:

1. To prepare themselves for singing.

2. To take a breath before starting, thus singing on the breath. The breath already existing into the lungs must be used first, then replaced by a new supply. This establishes a natural rhythm of breathing.

3. To attack the tone by a stroke (stroke of glottis). It must commence exactly as in talking.

4. To sing double vowels, like Ma-a, Me-e, Mi-i, Mo-o, Mu-u. In doing this the second vowel will always be dragged back into the throat by the tongue.

5. To accentuate the top notes, or the last of the exercises. This is done by most students. The tones must all be perfectly equal and colorless from the first to the last exercise.

Once pupils have acquired a certain freedom and dexterity in doing these exercises with the consonants B, M, L, they must practice all the other consonants of the alphabet. Thereafter start to use the syllables La, Le, Li, Lo, Lu, in alternation with the vowels alone, A—E—I—O—U in staccato form, until their experience in placing the voice is completely assured.

The above suggestions, besides being a valuable guide in placing the voice, can correct almost any defect in voice production, and establish the proper vocal mechanism for beginners.

In order to acquire the full command of a correct

voice production, available for all styles of music, pupils must enter into the practice of sustained tones—the most difficult achievement in the art of good singing—only after a perfect control of the staccato tones has been attained, and in the beginning they must be attempted only in combination with staccato tones. This constitutes the second series of exercises.

The third series is made up of only sustained tones, which, when produced correctly, commences to take on all the musical characteristics of the singing voice: volume, color, expression, which gradually develop the pupils' personal style of singing.

FACSIMILE OF MS. COPIED BY CARUSO HIMSELF AND CONTAINING HIS
ORIGINAL METHOD OF TEACHING HIMSELF HOW TO SING IN ENGLISH

Before going into the vocal exercises of The Scientific Culture of Voice it may be of interest to study closely an original manuscript written by Caruso himself as an aid in studying.

The importance given by Caruso to his enunciation in singing is shown by the care with which he translated into English the front page of this Neapolitan song, spelling the English version according to the Italian rules.

The handwriting of both the music and the words is his own, and the underscored words represent the English pronunciation "Italianized."

This series of staccato exercises is suggested for the purpose of making students attain the correct enunciation of their words as the best means for placing the singing voice through the proper formation of the speaking voice.

When once the voice is placed, by the means of the consonants, these same exercises must be practiced again by using the vowels A, E, I, O, U alone, in staccato form.

The vowels are more difficult to place, therefore in singing them alone particular care must be taken to enunciate them as they are enunciated when connected with consonants as, for instance, la, le, li, lo, lu. It would be a good practice at the beginning to alternate, la, le, li, lo, lu with a, e, i, o, u.

*VOCAL EXERCISES

FOR USE IN CONJUNCTION WITH

"THE SCIENTIFIC CULTURE OF THE 'VOICE"

In singing all the exercises which follow, the singer must strive to use the correct Italian pronunciation of the vowels and consonants.

FIRST SERIES - EXERCISE I^A

This exercise starts on C, using the major triad, descending four semi-tones; then on D♭ descending in the same manner; then on D, E♭ and E, descending on the latter nine semitones to and including G below the treble staff.

VOCAL EXERCISES (Cont'd)

FIRST SERIES - EXERCISE I^B

Major triad beginning on dominant (G), followed by same triad on tonic (C); then ascending by semitones with same figure from A♭ to F; then descending by same figure reversed to G below treble staff.

When correct voice production has been attained in each of the fore-going exercises with the consonants M, B, L, practice each of them with every consonant of the alphabet: for example

Ta, Te, Ti, To, Tu

Sa, Se, Si, So, Su

taking special care to articulate them properly

VOCAL EXERCISES (Cont'd)

FIRST SERIES - EXERCISE 2ᴬ

Ascending and descending the scale, starting on the tonic (C) and ending on the dominant (G), descending four semitones, then starting on Db and descending in same manner, then on D, Eb, and E, descending in last instance a full octave to E below the staff.

VOCAL EXERCISES (Cont'd)

FIRST SERIES - EXERCISE 2^B

Major scale starting on dominant (G) ascending and descending a fifth; then on tonic (C) in same manner; then a major third below (Ab) ascending to Eb, and descending in same way progressively to E below the staff.

VOCAL EXERCISES (Cont'd)

FIRST SERIES – EXERCISE 2ᶜ

la le li lo lu lo lo lo la

la le li lo lu lo lo lo la

la le li lo lu lo lo lo la

la le li lo, lu lo lo lo la

la le li lo lu lo lo lo la

la le li lo lu lo lo lo la etc.

etc.

After thoroughly practising this exercise with the syllables la, le, li, lo, lu, work with the other consonants of the alphabet, for example

Ba, Be, Bi, Bo, Bu

Ma, Me, Mi, Mo, Mu

Sa, Se, Si, So, Su etc.

Pronounce every syllable distinctly and clearly – this is one of the most important features in connection with the exercise.

VOCAL EXERCISES (Cont'd)

FIRST SERIES - EXERCISE 3

After practising these exercises by singing the syllable Lo on the top and descending notes, having acquired their correct production, the syllables La, Le, Li, Lo, Lu must be substituted and practised in place of Lo.

VOCAL EXERCISES (Cont'd)

FIRST SERIES - EXERCISE 4

Tempo moderato

La la la lo lo lo la   la la la lo lo lo la

la la la lo lo lo la   la la la lo lo lo la

la la la lo lo lo la   la la la lo lo lo la

etc.

etc.

When the correct production of this exercise is acquired, change the syllable on the top and descending notes, as in exercise 3.

VOCAL EXERCISES (Cont'd)

FIRST SERIES- EXERCISE 5

When the correct production of this exercise is acquired, change the syllable on the top and descending notes, as in exercise 3

292

VOCAL EXERCISES (Cont'd)

FIRST SERIES – EXERCISE 6

When the correct production of this exercise is acquired, change the syllable on the top and descending notes as in Exercise 3

VOCAL EXERCISES (Cont'd)

FIRST SERIES-- EXERCISE 7

Tempo moderato

la la lo lo lo lo   la   la lo lo lo lo   la   la lo lo lo lo   la

la -la lo lo lo lo   la   la la lo lo lo   la   la la lo lo lo   la

la la lo lo lo lo   la la la lo lo lo   la la la lo lo lo   la   *etc.*

etc.

When the correct production of this exercise is acquired, change the syllable on the top and descending notes as in Exercise 3

VOCAL EXERCISES (Cont'd)

FÍRST SERIES – EXERCISE 8

la la la la lo lo lo · lo lo lo lo lo la

la la la la lo lo lo lo lo lo lo lo la

la la la la lo lo lo. lo lo lo lo lo la

etc.

etc.

Continue Exercise 8 as in Exercise 2A, also in same manner as Exercise 2B and 2C. Voice production must be equal in volume and quality in every passage, and pronunciation must be perfect or voice will be misplaced. Also change syllables on top and descending notes as in Exercise 3

VOCAL EXERCISES (Cont'd)

FIRST SERIES – EXERCISE 9

Use the least amount of breath possible in order to become accustomed to its proper distribution. After each passage breathe deeply, and do not begin the next passage before complete relaxation is obtained.

When the correct production of this exercise is acquired, change the syllable on the top and descending notes as in Exercise 3

VOCAL EXERCISES (Cont'd)

SECOND SERIES- EXERCISE 1

Tempo moderato

la la la lo— lo lo lo lo lo la—   la la la lo— lo lo lo lo lo

la —   la la la lo— lo lo lo lo lo la —   la la la lo— lo

lo lo lo lo la —   la la la lo— lo .lo lo lo lo la—   etc.

etc.

VOCAL EXERCISES (Cont'd)

SECOND SERIES – EXERCISE 2

VOCAL EXERCISES (Cont'd)

SECOND SERIES – EXERCISE 3

Tempo moderato

la la la la lo ___ lo lo lo lo lo lo lo la

la la la la lo ___ lo lo lo lo lo lo lo la

la la la la lo ___ lo lo lo lo lo lo lo la   etc.

etc.

Practice this exercise in same order of transposition as that given in Exercises
2ᵃ, 2ᵇ, and 2ᶜ (First Series)

When the correct production is acquired, change the syllable on the top and de‧
scending notes as in Exercise 3 (First Series)

VOCAL EXERCISES (Cont'd)

SECOND SERIES - EXERCISE 4

In practicing this exercise, care must be taken that on the syllable de the tongue be completely relaxed between the teeth and left there until the next bar begins.

VOCAL EXERCISES (Cont'd)

SECOND SERIES - EXERCISE 5

Continue this exercise, ascending first to A below the staff up to and including C below the staff.

VOCAL EXERCISES (Cont'd)

THIRD SERIES - EXERCISE 1
SUSTAINED TONES

Continue this exercise up to C above Middle C and descend to the starting point. The preceding exercises of the first and second series must be practiced with sustained tones as in the above exercise.

CONCLUSION

A WORD FROM A LARYNGOLOGIST TO SINGERS

MANY books on *voice* and *voice culture,* written by singing teachers, assume almost the proportions of a Treaty on Physical Culture or on Laryngology by prescribing a large number of physical exercises or by dispensing advice of a purely medical character regarding the hygiene of the voice and the care of the throat.

As a laryngologist of many years' practice, mostly among professional singers, we cannot refrain— before closing this book—from having our say on these medical recommendations, coming for the most part from outsiders to the profession.

To the question, What measures of prevention against impairing the voice or what particular precautions for the throat must be taken by singers, we have only one emphatic reply, *Correct singing,* above all things.

It may seem an exaggerated and severe statement, but it is nevertheless true that in the majority of cases when singers complain about their throat and voice, their troubles cannot be ascribed to any disease, but are the direct result of a wrong voice production, the real source of worry for professional singers. "I have caught a bad cold" is the ready excuse to which a bad singer usually resorts, and which the public always accepts, while the experienced laryngologist easily finds out that the "cold" is nothing but habitual strain on the vocal organs.

We may quote here the case of a coloratura soprano, whom we kept warning for years, when she called on us for treatment—usually after performances or recitals—that there was nothing wrong with her throat, except the strain of bad singing. At last one day she became convinced that she should change her method of singing and acquire an easier voice production. She has never had to consult a throat specialist since then and her habitual after-performance colds have completely disappeared. Of course, like all ordinary mortals, singers are liable to suffer from colds and sore throats, and so far science has not discovered any special means to render them immune. In order to guard against these indispositions they must comport themselves as any intelligent person does.

Singing does affect the throat, but *bad singing* sets in a chronic congestion of the vocal organs through undue strain and violent effort, just as correct dancing does not harm the legs, while bad dancing may deform or sprain the ankles or even cripple the performer.

In a previous chapter we have already stated that a strongly developed breathing apparatus or throat is not always a determining factor in good singing, but that correct voice production greatly contributes to the muscular strengthening of these organs. The physical constitution of a singer is independent of his natural or inherited gift for the art, and the physical training which is indispensable in the case of a prize fighter or an acrobat is of no avail for the development of the vocal organs; some great artists are and have been small and thin, some others of lesser fame are or have been, on the contrary, endowed with an exceptional *embonpoint*, and, so far, it has been impossible to measure talent by inches or by pounds.

The general health condition of an artist has certainly much to do with his singing, but this is true with the proper discharge of duties in any other walk of life.

There are hygienic principles which govern all the physiological functions of our system, whether they be of a more muscular nature, like boxing, fencing, and other sports, or more subject to psychological control, like painting, playing, singing, etc.

For the proper performance of our work, in both instances, we need the assistance of hygienic rules, so that our system may be kept in a high degree of physiological efficiency; but there is a difference in the hygienic rules pertaining to each of the above cases. While it is urgent for a boxer or a fencer to keep his muscles in continual training, it is hardly necessary for a thinker, a writer, or anybody who is devoted to a purely intellectual form of activity to overtax his physical strength. As singing belongs to this latter class of activities, all books and methods advocating physical training for singers seem to consider singing more as a muscular action than as an intellectual achievement.

We would suggest that singers take care of their health just by following the normal rules of all intelligent people, without exerting themselves in any form of physical training. The vocal apparatus is a delicate machine, and must be treated carefully and gently; general health is its best support.

There are no medicinal preparations of any kind that ought to be recommended to singers who are in normal health; the beauty of their voice cannot be enhanced or preserved by doctor's prescriptions.

We cannot deny that the organs we make most use of in our daily occupation are our weakest spots, more readily exposed to the attack of adverse conditions. It is true, in the case of most singers, that their vocal organs are more sensitive than the others to exposure or climatic variations. No pharmaceutical products, however, can bring a radical relief in such cases; singers who are compelled by their profession to migrate from warm lands to cold countries, from dry climates to damp climates, must try and acclimatize themselves by contracting open-air habits, by avoiding overheated rooms, as well as cold and damp habitations; they must lead a regular, wholesome life, because a profession that is exercised mostly late at night taxes more our vital resources than work done earlier in the day.

Moderation must be the guiding rule: cold baths, cold applications to the outside of the throat for a few minutes in the morning, followed by a light massage of the neck to promote circulation; but, above all, a daily practice of vocal exercises of light nature, which act as an internal massage on the vocal organs. These exercises must be done often during the day, for fifteen or twenty minutes at a time. There is no more danger to the vocal organs in practicing even several hours a day, if the voice production is correct, than there is to the fingers of a pianist or a violinist, though some allowance must be made for the vocal organs, made of delicate tissues, which must be used with more care than the hardened muscles of our fingers.

Here again—in closing our book—we cannot refrain from mentioning Caruso as the most wonderful rebuke of all the prejudices and the antiquated rules that still govern to-day's schools of voice culture. The great artist was a heavy smoker and indulged in liberties that the majority of singers would consider as forbidden fruit.

We have never known him to use any special preparations or to take such precautions as any ordinary mortal would not take. A light salt solution was his usual gargle during the performances, and when his throat was much congested—often on account of smoking—he used a spray of *apothesine* and *adrenalin,* prescribed by us. But the great singer was more fond of munching an apple between acts than of anything else.

He was as simple in his living as in his hygienic habits, when his vocal organs were concerned. Alas, his premature death shows us now that he was perhaps over-generous with his own vitality, and that on the altar of Art he laid down his life as a sublime sacrifice.

His tragic death evokes in our memory the beautiful words that the great French poet—Alfred de Musset—wrote almost eighty years ago, at the death of Malibran, another great singer:

Ce qu'il nous faut pleurer sur ta tombe hâtive
Ce n'est pas l'art divin, ni ses savants secrets:
Quelque autre étudiera cet art que tu créais;
C'est ton âme, CARUSO, et ta grandeur naïve,
C'est cette voix du cœur qui seule au cœur arrive,
Que nul autre, après toi, ne nous rendra jamais.

(1)

Lightning Source UK Ltd.
Milton Keynes UK
12 July 2010

156900UK00002B/5/P

9 781443 756457